The Beautiful People
and
Other Aggravations

The Beautiful People
and
Other Aggravations

Rose Madeline Mula

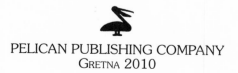

PELICAN PUBLISHING COMPANY
GRETNA 2010

The word "Pelican" and the depiction of a pelican
are trademarks of Pelican Publishing Company, Inc.,
and are registered in the U.S. Patent and Trademark Office.

Library of Congress Cataloging-in-Publication Data

Mula, Rose Madeline.
  The beautiful people and other aggravations / Rose Madeline Mula.
      p. cm.
  ISBN 978-1-58980-688-7 (pbk. : alk. paper) 1. American wit and
humor. I. Title.
  PN6162.M73 2010
  818'.5407—dc22

                                        2009053946

Printed in the United States of America
Published by Pelican Publishing Company, Inc.
1000 Burmaster Street, Gretna, Louisiana 70053

To the Davis Five:
Shelley, Jack, Madeline,
Alexandra, and Jonathan, with all my love

Contents

The Beautiful People
and
Other Aggravations

The Beautiful People

It's just not fair. I try to be a good sport. I really do.

Even though the only exotic sites I see these days are on PBS travelogues, I don't complain when those who are not as financially challenged as I winter in the Greek Islands, summer in their palatial digs in the Hamptons, and jet off to Paris for a weekend whenever they have a hankering to nibble on a croissant at a sidewalk *patisserie* on the Rue de la Paix.

Furthermore, no one hears me whine (much) because everyone else on the planet has cable TV or satellite dishes that pull in more than five hundred channels sharply and clearly, while I have to keep adjusting my rabbit ears to decrease the "snow" on the half-dozen network channels I can coax in. Neither do I bellyache that I have to watch those stations on an old, bulky nineteen-inch set instead of a state-of-the-art sixty-inch plasma wall display.

And my Wal-Mart radio may not sound as if I have a symphony orchestra in my living room, but I'm sure my neighbors appreciate that I'm not drowning out their own sophisticated, surround-sound music systems.

As for all the walkers and joggers I meet at the local track, I try not to envy the thousand songs they can choose from on their cute, tiny iPods. I tell myself that I'm glad I don't have to go through the hassle of downloading and cataloging all those tunes. Besides, the cassette in my Walkman provides me with more than enough music to power my daily two-mile trek.

At least I have a computer. So what if I can't afford DSL or broadband and still have only a slow dial-up connection to the Internet that ties up my phone whenever I'm online? Actually, that's a blessing; because when hoity-toity socialites don't call to invite me to their A-list bashes or publishers and producers aren't ringing and clamoring for my services, I can tell myself it's simply because my phone is busy and they can't reach me.

I don't even grumble when I have to push my vacuum cleaner around myself because all the Merry Maids in town are busy doing the housework for those who can actually pay them (which explains why they're so merry).

But it's gone too far. Now not only do the beautiful people lead more glamorous, less stressful lives than I, but they're all becoming even *more* beautiful because they can pay exorbitant fees for face lifts, tummy tucks, Botox, liposuction, collagen injections, implants (breast, hair, and dental), and more.

Soon nursing homes and retirement communities will be filled with gorgeous, smooth-faced men and women in wheelchairs or tottering around on canes or walkers.

Unless I hit the lottery and can also indulge in multiple cosmetic surgeries, before long I'm going to be the only person in America who looks her age—which means I'll look older than the few women still alive who are old enough to be my mother.

Some deride those who they say have had too much "work" done—people whose faces are so unnaturally tight they no longer have any expression whatsoever. So? What's so terrible about that? I would *kill* for that look!

But how to get it? I'm tempted to hit the streets carrying a large sign that proclaims, WILL WORK FOR BOTOX.

Meanwhile, I'll just keep slathering on the drugstore wrinkle-decrease cream. Yeah, right—that's going to work.

The Stranger in My Mirror

A very weird thing has happened. A strange old lady has moved into my house. I have no idea who she is, where she came from, or how she got in. I certainly didn't invite her. All I know is that one day she wasn't there, and the next day she was.

She's very clever. She manages to keep out of sight for the most part; but whenever I pass a mirror, I catch a glimpse of her there; and when I look into a mirror directly to check on my appearance, suddenly she's hogging the whole thing, completely obliterating my gorgeous face and body. It's very disconcerting. I've tried screaming at her to leave—but she just screams back, grimacing horribly. She's really rather frightening.

If she's going to hang around, the least she could do is offer to pay rent. But no. Every once in a while I do find a couple of dollar bills on the kitchen counter, or some loose change on my bureau or on the floor; but that certainly isn't enough. In fact, though I don't like to jump to conclusions, I think she steals money from me quite regularly. I go to the ATM and withdraw one hundred dollars, and a few days later, it's gone. I certainly don't go through it that fast, so I can only conclude that the old lady pilfers it. You'd think she'd spend some of it on wrinkle cream. God knows she needs it.

Money isn't the only thing she's taking; food seems to disappear at an alarming rate. Especially the good stuff—ice cream, cookies, candy . . . I just can't seem to keep them in the house. She really has a sweet tooth. She should watch it; she's putting on the pounds. I think she realizes that; and to make herself feel better, I know she's tampering with my scale so I'll think that I'm gaining weight, too. For an old lady, she's really quite childish. She also gets into my closets when I'm not home and alters all my clothes. They're getting tighter every day.

Another thing: I wish she'd stop messing with my files and the papers on my desk. I can't find a thing any more. This is particularly hard to deal with because I'm extremely neat and organized; however, she manages to jumble everything up so nothing is where it's supposed to be. Furthermore, when I program my VCR to tape something important, she fiddles with it after I leave the room so it records the wrong channel or shuts off completely.

She finds innumerable, imaginative ways to irritate me. She gets to my newspapers, magazines, and mail before me and blurs all the print; and she's done something sinister with the volume controls on my TV, radio, and phone. Now all I hear are mumbles and whispers. She's also made my stairs steeper, my vacuum cleaner heavier, all my knobs and faucets hard to turn, and my bed higher and a real challenge to climb into and out of. Moreover, she gets to my groceries as soon as I shelve them and applies super glue to the tops of every jar and bottle so they're just about impossible to open. Is this any way to repay my hospitality?

I don't even get any respite at night. More than once her snoring has awakened me. I don't know why she can't do something about that. It's very unattractive.

As if all this isn't bad enough, she is no longer confining her malevolence to the house. She's now found a way to sneak into my car with me and follow me wherever I go. I see her reflection in store windows as I pass, and she's taken all the fun out of clothes shopping because her penchant for monopolizing mirrors has extended to dressing rooms. When I try something on, she dons an identical outfit—which looks ridiculous on her—and then stands directly in front of me so I can't see how great it looks on me.

I thought she couldn't get any meaner than that, but yesterday she proved me wrong. She had the nerve to come with me when I went to have some passport pictures taken, and she actually stepped in front of the camera just as the shutter clicked. Disaster! I have never seen such a terrible picture. How can I go abroad now? No customs official is ever going to believe that that crone scowling from my passport is me.

She's walking on very thin ice. If she keeps this up, I swear I'll put her in a home. On second thought, I shouldn't be too hasty. First, I think I'll check with the IRS and see if I can claim her as a dependent.

The Curse of the Purse

What is it with women's pocketbooks? Who decrees that their dimensions and style must change from year to year, season to season? And why do we care what "who" says anyway? Why do we slavishly follow "who's" dictates?

It's ridiculous.

A few years ago, fashion determined that our purses must be tiny or, at the very least, small. The clutch was in. Practicality was out. Unless a woman's other accessory was a man with many pockets that could hold her necessities, she was limited to making do with a lipstick, one tissue, and a credit card. No cash. Not even a single bill. Because if she bought something that required change, she'd have no room for it. If she needed to carry reading glasses, or maybe an extra tampon, she was out of luck.

Today, on the other hand, the clutch is out and the minisuitcase is *de rigueur*. Bags so huge and heavy, even when empty, they should be on wheels. Bags with a myriad of gleaming brass buckles, studs, decorative chains, and enough inner and outer pockets to accommodate a cell phone, a Blackberry, a Palm Pilot, an address book (in case the Palm Pilot's batteries expire), a GPS system, a digital camera, a checkbook, a calculator, sun glasses, a memo pad, a pen, a toothbrush, dental floss, not one but several lipsticks, eye shadow, mascara, blush, powder, concealer, a pack of tissues, nail polish, a can of Mace, extra car and house keys, a book (hey, you have to have something to do while standing in those lines at the supermarket, bank, and post office), an iPod, hair brush, hair spray, mirror, hand lotion, a water bottle, a collapsible umbrella, your computer's memory stick with your back-up documents (can't leave it home where a fire could possibly destroy it, along with your computer), and, of course, a wallet bulging with a driver's license, cash, a dozen credit cards, ATM card, library card, medical insurance cards, auto club ID, recent pictures of your kids, baby pictures of your kids, pictures of your current husband/boyfriend/partner, pictures of all your exes—just for starters, plus a granola bar to give you the energy required to tote all that stuff.

The irony is that despite (or because of) the bags' multiple compartments designed to keep things organized, you can never remember where you put what. You end up unzipping, unsnapping, and unbuckling them all before you find the item you need. Then, naturally, there are the objects that have no designated compartments. Things like that half a roll of Tums, a band aid, tea bag, coupons, pill box, a crumpled grocery list, all of which drift to Never Never Land—the bottom of the bag— where they are lost forever.

Another problem with those oversized purses is where do you keep them? Especially if you have the multiple purses fashion mandates—summer and winter bags in various colors to match your thirty pairs of shoes. You certainly can't tuck them into a dresser drawer. And forget the floor of your closet. All those shoes are there, remember? If the huge pocketbook trend continues, new homes will offer purse storage rooms, in addition to walk-in closets; and automobiles will have to add special overhead bins, like on airplanes, to stow our purses.

We used to get along without carrying all those so-called necessities with us wherever we went. Why can we no longer manage without them? Certainly, we could, but the problem is that nature abhors a vacuum. The larger the bag, the stronger the compulsion to fill every centimeter of space.

It's the same principle that applies to homes: the more space, the more stuff we cram into it. If, for example, we move from a five-hundred-square-foot studio apartment (which holds all the possessions we need to live a full life) to a ten-thousand-square-foot mansion, I guarantee that within two weeks, every room and closet, as well as all the storage space in the cellar/attic/garage (none of which we had in the studio), will be bulging with miscellany we suddenly must have. If the space is there, whether in our homes or in our purses, we're compelled to fill it.

We can only hope, therefore, that pocketbook designers will have pity on us and not foist even larger bags on us. If they do, we may then feel we must carry a roll of paper towels and/or toilet tissue, a bottle of salad dressing, a sandwich, a portable DVD player, an extra pair of shoes . . . where will it all end?

It used to be that the only thing we were cautioned not to leave home without was our American Express card.

Ah, those were the days!

How Great to See You!
You Look Marvelous!

I'm depressed. I just returned from the first high-school reunion I ever attended. I refuse to say which one. Not which high school—which year. I don't want anyone to know. I won't even admit it to myself.

What I will tell you is that none of my classmates showed up. They sent their grandparents instead, all of who insisted they had gone to school with me. No way. I could not relate to those people. They were white-haired or bald, fat or frail, stooped and lame. None of them bore the slightest resemblance to the yearbook pictures reproduced on their nametags. (Whose fiendish idea was that?!) That's what clinched it—proved they were frauds.

I, on the other hand, look exactly the same as I did back then. Well, almost, except for a few interesting character lines that only enhance my youthful charm. In fact, all the elderly people I talked with gasped when I told them my name. They all reacted the same way, their gazes shifting in disbelief from my face to my yearbook picture on my nametag. Obviously, they were astonished at how little I've changed. Nothing else could explain their incredulity.

Of course, I tried to be kind and commented on how well the years had treated them. I didn't consider such flattery to be lies but, rather, acts of mercy. Poor things. God knows they can't often hear that. To be truthful, I don't hear it much myself. I'm sure people compliment me all the time (after all, how could they not?), but they mumble so badly that they're hard to understand.

My girl friend Jeannie was at the reunion. (That's right, I said "girl" friend. Females of my generation never refer to ourselves as "women.") Jeannie couldn't wait to see Frank, the handsome hunk we had all swooned over in high school. (Yes, in those days, we swooned—do I hear you snickering? That's very rude.) I had bumped into him earlier. I pointed him out to her.

"That's Frank, over there; the one with the walker."

Jeannie gasped. "He's old!"

Well, duh! What did she expect? Frank is wrinkled; his once lean body has turned into cookie dough; and his teeth click when he talks. At least he doesn't have white hair. He doesn't have *any* hair.

When Jeannie recovered from her initial shock, she gamely approached him to reintroduce herself.

"Frank! You're as handsome as ever!" she gushed.

(Yeah, we used to gush, as well as swoon.)

"Why, thank you!" beamed Frank, the old twinkle returning to his eyes for a moment. "I'd like you to meet my granddaughter," he said, calling a lovely lass to his side.

Jeannie turned to her, "Your grandfather used to be so cute," she gushed again. Frank stopped beaming. "Used to be?" he croaked. "Whatever happened to 'as handsome as ever?'"

"Excuse me," said Jeannie, trying to extract her foot from her mouth, "I just spotted Andy Harrington over there. I went to the junior prom with him! I'm going over to say hello."

I didn't have the heart to tell her that Andy was the feeble geezer clutching the bar to keep from falling. The guy she was rushing toward was a teenaged bus boy.

As I was trying to restore Frank's wounded pride, another of the elderly party crashers approached me, squinting at my nametag.

"I remember you," he said, "you were in my typing class."

"No," I said, "I never took typing in high school."

"Yeah, you did," he insisted, miffed.

And he shuffled away to squint at another woman's nametag. Maybe it was just a clever ploy to stare at bosoms. On second thought, there wasn't a bosom in the room worth staring at, other than mine; but I'm much too modest to mention that.

Just then, the pianist the reunion committee had hired started tickling the ivories—"As Time Goes By," "Those Were the Days," "Silver Threads Among the Gold." He had an endless repertoire of melancholy melodies.

I had a sudden yearning for heavy metal or rap, even though I hate them. As he played, a few couples teetered across the floor, holding each other up, apparently trying to pretend they were back in the old crepe-paper-decorated gymnasium.

After an hour or so of this charade, the MC mercifully asked everyone to please be seated. Dinner was about to be served. I prayed that the meal wouldn't consist of soup, puréed veggies, and Jell-O. On the other hand, if it was solid food, I worried about how most of the group would deal with it. It would not be pretty. I hoped a contingent of EMTs was standing by.

I vowed never to attend another reunion.

Three's a Crowd
(A Tale of Second Childhood)

My small condo is getting much too crowded. I had become accustomed to living alone, and I enjoyed my freedom and independence. But now I have two uninvited houseguests.

The first one to move in without my permission a few years ago was an old lady who didn't even have the courtesy to introduce herself to me and who never speaks to me. The ugly crone simply lurks in my mirrors and generally makes my life miserable. She's very sadistic and enjoys inflicting pain in all my joints.

As if that weren't bad enough, my living situation has now become even more intolerable. A bratty kid has also invaded my home. Unlike the old lady, this new resident is completely invisible. I never see her or her reflection anywhere, but she's here all right.

She leaves chewy caramels around even though she knows I can't resist them. I'm sure she hopes a few teeth will fall out so the tooth fairy will visit and leave shiny quarters, which she, of course, will steal before I wake up—that is, if I ever fall asleep. You see, she has also somehow irritated the sandman so much that he almost never visits any more. She's delighted about that, because when I can't sleep, I get out of bed and go into the den and turn on the computer, which she then appropriates. Instead of letting me answer my e-mail, write an article, or do some research, she snatches the mouse and clicks onto Solitaire or Hearts. I have absolutely no control over her. She plays those stupid games until 3:00 or 4:00 A.M. before she lets me turn off the computer and go back to bed.

She also likes noncomputer games and toys and has confiscated a good chunk of my limited closet space to house her collection. When friends with children visit, she hauls out her cache and insists I join in the games instead of conversing with the adults. Therefore, I'm stuck playing Candy Land or Go Fish while the grown-ups get to discuss stimulating topics such as the fluctuation of the peseta or whatever happened to aluminum Christmas trees. It's just not fair.

The holidays are particularly stressful since the kid has arrived. On New Year's Eve, because she's too young to be allowed into the glamorous night spots to which I receive a myriad of invitations, she won't let me go. No, I have to stay home with her and watch that ridiculous ball drop in Times Square.

On February 14, I don't receive a single valentine. I used to get dozens! I'm sure the kid intercepts the mailman and confiscates them. What other possible explanation can there be? She even destroys the cards the old lady insists her beaus still send. The kid thinks "beaus" is a funny word; and she says the old lady lies when she claims she ever had any. You can't imagine the ruckus this causes between the two of them! I'm tired of acting as referee.

Then there's April Fool's Day. I swear I'll disconnect the phone if the kid doesn't stop calling tobacco shops and asking if they have Prince Albert in the can. I blame the old lady for teaching her that ancient prank. They either bicker or get into mischief together. I don't know which is worse.

On Easter, the old lady insists that the kid put on a new hat and go to church, but the kid prefers to stay home and hunt for colored eggs and chocolate bunnies. More fighting.

The kid also loves Halloween. Even though I tell her that now that I'm in a condo building no children ever come trick or treating, she insists on stockpiling candy, just in case. Naturally, it's always all left over. For days afterwards, she force-feeds all those caloric goodies to me.

At Christmas, she whines because I refuse to take her to see

Santa Claus. I tell her she's not a baby any more and it's time she stopped believing in that myth. Nevertheless, she never fails to hang a stocking every Christmas Eve. Of course, it's empty in the morning, which makes her very depressed with longing for the good old days. How does she know about the good old days? Our roommate, the old lady, keeps telling her about them—ad nauseum. I, for one, am very sick of hearing those same stories over and over again.

She's also claimed the TV as her own. She's very immature, even for a kid. She's hopelessly addicted to sitcoms. I want to watch something uplifting and educational, but no! She insists on having her way; and since she always gets to the remote before I do (the old lady hides it, and the kid is always the first to find it), I can do nothing but watch her idiotic shows with her. My brain is turning to mush.

Speaking of mush, her food preferences are abominable. Vegetables? Forget it. She makes such a scene at the supermarket whenever I approach the produce section that I have no choice but to allow her to drag me down the cookie aisle, the deli counter for the richest cheeses she can find, the take-out department for pepperoni pizza, and the freezer for double-fudge ice cream. I try to talk her into settling for sorbet, but she makes a dreadful face and starts screaming. What can I do? If I slap her and pull her away, I'll be arrested for child abuse. Though I'm delighted when she finally agrees to leave the market, I dread the confrontation that I know awaits us at home. The minute we get inside the door, the old lady starts rummaging through the bags for her bran cereal. Believe me; she is not thrilled when all she finds is sugar frosted flakes.

I keep reading about the problems of "the sandwich generation"— those who must care for elderly relatives and children. It's a real challenge. I now know from experience. What I don't know is how it happened to me. Unfortunately, my parents are gone, and I never had children. So how did I fall into the sandwich trap?

It's a puzzle, but I don't have time to figure it out right now. I have to call a locksmith to add a few more deadbolts before anyone else moves in.

Aiding and Abetting

Do you worry about a burglar breaking into your home and stealing your precious possessions? Have you a favorite hiding place for valuables?

No, not the ice cube trays in the freezer. Every self-respecting thief knows that one. There are so many other very clever ways to conceal your priceless gems, credit cards, laptops, and the money you're trying to hide from the IRS. Just last week, I read a magazine article that detailed dozens of extremely unlikely possibilities where you can stash your cache—places where a burglar would never dream to look.

Unless, of course, said burglar read the same article.

I would describe some of these hiding places for you here, but, like the writer of the aforementioned magazine piece, I would be aiding and abetting potential thieves. Not that they can't find the information for themselves; but they should at least have to work for it.

If all robbers were illiterate, no problem. Unfortunately, however, odds are that your friendly neighborhood thief made it past the first grade and can read and most likely even has computer skills that enable him to log on to Google on his stolen laptop and access not only the magazine article I mentioned but thousands of others on the same subject.

Either that, or he can just wait for the postman to deliver his daily pile of miscellany that is sure to include at least a couple of mail order catalogues—which, in turn, have ads for fake bricks, flower pots with false bottoms, hollow picture frames, faux soup cans, and other items suitable for concealing small treasures.

OOOPS! I just helped a burglar somewhere, didn't I?

However, these concerns are relatively minor.

Even more disturbing these days are news articles that fuel the imaginations of terrorists. Often I read things like "Authorities are concerned that Titanic Towers in Metropolis is particularly susceptible to terrorist attack because of its unstable structural design and easy access to its rooftop." Or, "Five hundred thousand fans are expected to fill XYZ Stadium to capacity for the championship game on Saturday, raising fears that a handful of suicide bombers could cause extensive fatalities." And I cringe when government officials tell us to go about our business and to storm the shopping malls in droves but to keep a watchful eye for "suspicious activity." (I can hear a potential fanatic saying, "Ooooh! Shopping malls! I hadn't thought about that!")

I know, I know. The bad guys are already aware of our vulnerabilities, but maybe they haven't considered one or two possibilities. Do we have to provide them with a detailed "To Do" list?

And once we've helped terrorists identify potential targets, we go even further: We actually give them recipes for constructing bombs. Honest. I've seen them in the daily newspaper. Again, I'm sure Google is a gateway to a treasure trove of destructive "How-Tos." I have yet to find a simple, fail-proof recipe for lemon meringue pie on the site, but I bet I'd have no trouble whatsoever researching the exact ingredients and proportions for something that goes BOOM! and wreaks havoc. To be honest, I haven't checked this out because I'm afraid Big Brother may be monitoring my Internet searches; and the FBI would come and break down my door before I even logged off. Me, a perfectly innocent, mature (okay, old) woman they'd cart off to a high-security jail; but if a wild-eyed young man named Mohammed with a history of violence conducted a similar Internet search, the law would leave him alone. God forbid they should be accused of racial profiling.

I'm also certain that all the ingredients for manufacturing explosive devices are readily available at any hardware store or garden supply center. A young person might need to show ID to purchase cigarettes in America, but he would have no problem at all acquiring everything needed to assemble a horde of weapons of mass destruction. I suppose it's comforting to know that while some kid could be planning mayhem and multiple murders, at least his lungs are clear, and he won't be subjecting anyone to secondhand smoke.

What else are we doing to make things easy for the baddies?

I wouldn't be surprised to find books titled *Terrorism for Dummies* and *Burglary Made Easy* featured on Amazon.com.

Would you check please? I'd do it, but I can't afford to arouse suspicion. I think I'm under surveillance since I tried to sneak nine items through the "Eight Items or Fewer" checkout aisle at the market last week.

A Time to Be Born and a Time to Die

I'm painfully conscious of the fact that I have a more or less preordained expiration date. But since it's not stamped on my derrière or any other part of my anatomy (at least no part that's visible to me), I don't know what it is. Fortunately. I'd rather be surprised.

What about all those inanimate necessities we utilize daily. They also have circumscribed life spans that we should heed if we want to survive to our own maximum "Discard After" date.

Of course, everyone knows that medicines and drugs have very stringent expiration dates; and we all understand that most foods have a limited "Use By" date; but some data I recently read surprised me.

I did not realize, for instance, that once you open a can of coffee, it's good for only a month. Not great news. I drink instant for my daily breakfast. (I know, I know—that's so lowbrow; but what do you expect from someone who buys wine in a jug?) I brew perked coffee only for my monthly Scrabble group and occasional dinner guests, so a can of coffee lasts me at least six months.

As for wine, I do buy it in bottles occasionally to have on hand for company. I'm not so uncouth that I plunk a jug on the table during a dinner party. Au contraire, I keep my lovely wine rack fully stocked with stylish bottles to make a good impression, but apparently, that's not wise. I just learned that unopened bottled wine has a shelf life of only three years from its vintage date. Fine wines, on the other hand, last from twenty to one hundred years.

Since none of mine fits that latter category, I've got to have lots of company soon or start guzzling my cache myself.

Even chocolate has a limited shelf life—one year from the date of production, I'm told. For me that's not a problem. In my house, no piece of chocolate has ever survived longer than twenty-four hours after leaving the grocery bag or the hands of a gift giver.

I think I've always known that even canned goods have a limited life, but I believed that anything in a freezer should last forever. Not so. If you've been stashing TV dinners in there for a couple of years, along with that extra turkey you got from your boss the Thanksgiving before last, you'd better kiss them goodbye. No, wait! Your lips may freeze to them. Just toss them without a sentimental farewell.

And when did Aunt Matilda give you that fruitcake that's in the back right-hand corner? Wasn't it the Christmas that your college-graduate son was in sixth grade? Yes, they say fruitcake never spoils; but you'll never eat it. You've been saving it just to spare Aunt Matilda's feelings. Hello! She died two years ago. Even if she's looking down at you from a perch in Paradise, do you think she still cares about anything as mundane as her fruitcake?

Many other foods—far too numerous to itemize—are doomed to an early demise. Suffice it to say that if anything edible is older than the last New Year's resolution you broke, it probably should go.

And it isn't just food items that have short life spans. Recently I learned that many of the household and personal care products we use also have expiration dates, which may or may not be displayed on their packaging. These include air fresheners, dish and laundry detergents, furniture polish and other cleaning agents, most of which become obsolete even before your computer.

Take Windex, for instance. I was stunned to learn that it has only a two-year life. Considering how infrequently I wash windows, unless someone invents a Viagra for Windex, there's no way I'm going to use up that bottle before it loses its potency—which I assume is what happens after two years. Or possibly it suddenly explodes. Or maybe it just moves to a Windex-retirement community. I have no idea.

And did you know that bar soap is supposed to expire in eighteen months to three years? I still have half a dozen cakes of Ivory left from a stash I moved from my prior home eleven years ago—and I have no idea how long I had it before the move. I do have a vague recollection of stocking up at a big soap sale about twenty years ago. That was when I had a large cellar and tons of storage space. I now realize that having all those extra shelves and closets was not a big advantage.

Even deodorant should be tossed after two years. Oh, oh! That's right—it, too, was on special two decades ago. That's why that shoebox in my linen closet is brimful of sprays, roll-ons, and solids. (Hey, they were all on sale.)

And what about all those lipsticks we women (and some men, I'm sure) have tucked into our cosmetic bags and pocketbooks? Yes, they should also be replaced every couple of years. Of course, your favorite shade will no longer be manufactured then, but that's life. The same holds true for *all* makeup—foundation, mascara, eye shadow, blush, and all lotions and hair products as well. Do you think it's really true? Or, as in Mark Twain's case, are the reports of their early deaths greatly exaggerated?

Perfume, too, supposedly lasts only one to two years, I'm told. I still have a full bottle of Chanel No. 5 that I bought on my 1963 trip to Paris. I've been saving it for a special occasion. It's been over four decades and I still haven't opened the bottle. Apparently nothing important enough has come up yet. So much for my exciting life.

However, that's changing. I'm planning a very scintillating full day tomorrow. I'll be cleaning out my medicine cabinet, pantry, refrigerator, drawers, and my hoard of cosmetics—a very unusual activity for me. I suppose it could even be considered special.

Maybe I'll commemorate the occasion by dabbing on some of my 1963 Chanel.

Whatever Happened to . . .?

I sometimes feel I was born in a previous millennium. So many things I grew up with no longer exist.

Remember pin boys at bowling alleys, for example? Before automated pinsetters usurped their jobs, they sat on a perch at the end of the alley and then swooped down to replace any pins that had been knocked over. I was a rotten bowler; I made their job a snap. One reason I did so badly was that the cute pin boy made me self-conscious. The harder I tried to impress him, the worse my performance.

Speaking of cute boys, a big attraction at the movies back in my girlhood were the ushers in their tight navy blue jackets festooned with brass buttons and gold braid (I've always been a sucker for a uniform) who showed us to our seats in the palatial movie palaces of yore. Today, we fend for ourselves in stark, unadorned screening rooms. And when the ushers disappeared, they took with them the movie projectionists, who I often felt must have been very bored running the same film every day and evening for a week. Did I say "film"? I should have said "films" because every theatre always played a double feature. Today we see only one movie, powered by a robotic projector; and we no longer get any free dishes or cutlery with our tickets.

Joining those ushers and projectionists in the unemployment line are all the former strict housemothers at women's college dorms who would never allow a "gentleman caller" upstairs.

Today, coed dorms with unisex bathrooms are common; some schools also offer coed rooms. Is that crazy, or is it just me?

One thing I don't miss from the old days is luggage that you needed a forklift to haul up off the floor. How come we sent men to the moon before someone came up with the brilliant, but obvious, idea of wheels for suitcases?

Do you remember the cars of yesterday? All had running boards, some had rumble seats, and none had automatic transmission, power brakes, electric windows and door locks, cruise control, or power steering—parallel parking in a tight spot in those days took muscle. Cars back then didn't have electric turn signals either. You had to crank open your window and stick your hand out (in balmy weather, monsoons, or blizzards) to indicate that you were going to make a turn. The old Fords, Chevys, and Chryslers also didn't have heaters or defrosters. It was a tossup as to whether you'd succumb to frostbite before your windshield would freeze over. And in the dog days of summer no air conditioning. Just hot wind and exhaust fumes from passing cars blowing through your open windows. However, these inconveniences were offset by the fact that gas cost about fourteen cents per gallon.

If you were lucky enough to own a washing machine in the good old days, it had no spin cycle—just a hand-operated wringer that you fed the clothes through. No dryer. We hung our laundry, summer and winter, with wooden pins on something called a "line," a length of rope stretched from tree to tree in the backyard. If it rained on washday, we strung the wash on a line in the cellar, an unfinished basement, probably with a dirt floor. Downstairs playrooms, dens, or family rooms? Not back then. We didn't need them. We had no TVs or computers to accommodate. (How did we ever survive without CNN, Oprah, Leno, Google, MapQuest, e-mail?)

Telephones didn't have dials back then, and they didn't come in a myriad of styles and colors. Only one model, a clunky, black two-piece job with a mouthpiece mounted on a six-inch rod and a cord connected to an earpiece that hooked onto a lever near the top of the rod. To make a call, we picked up the earpiece and an operator would ask, "Number please?" and then connect us. Also, we spoke on a "party line," a connection that we shared with one or two other families. When we picked up the earpiece to make a call, if we heard others speaking, we were expected to hang up quietly and try again later. However, some people (not me, of course) would just pretend to hang up and, instead, would listen to the conversation. Who could blame us (I mean, them). We had no TV, no Internet, and no *National Enquirer.* Where else were we going to hear the gossip of the day?

Furthermore, everyone in the family made do with just one telephone (no extensions for every room); and that one phone had a wire that secured it firmly to its station. If anyone had told us that one day we would have cordless instruments in our homes—and that we'd even carry with us everywhere tiny portable, wireless phones (that could even take pictures!)—we would have called the men in the little white coats to come and whisk that kook away to the nearest asylum.

And whatever happened to girdles? Oh, wait—they're still with us, but today they're called "shapewear." Unfortunately, shapewear is just as uncomfortable as girdles.

Remember spring and fall cleaning? My mother used to dismantle every room in the house, twice a year, and disinfect, scrub, polish, and vacuum every inch of furniture, walls, floors, and fixtures and then change the curtains and bedspreads to complement the season. Does anyone still do that? I hate to admit it, but my beds and windows wear the same clothes year-round; and I shudder to think what may be hiding behind my cornices and under my sofas.

And whatever happened to propellers on planes, premicro-wave cooking, single-speed bicycles, galoshes, cloth diapers, typewriters, carbon paper, nondigital cameras and film, "Stella Dallas" and other radio serials, and songs with beautiful melodies and lovely lyrics you could actually understand?

I do know what happened to after-supper games of Red Rover and Kick the Can; they've been deposed by TV and computer games. News flash: Fiddling with a remote, keyboard, and mouse doesn't constitute aerobic exercise.

All these changes have come about in my lifetime. Granted, I'm not a kid; but, though some may disagree, I'm not ancient yet either. I can't imagine what the next fifty to one hundred years will bring. Old folks then will probably be reminiscing about their long-gone plasma TV sets, which most likely will have been replaced by three-dimensional systems that totally immerse viewers into the action, and their intercontinental jet tours, which will have been supplanted by interplanetary space travel.

I might even live to see it all since every day scientists are discovering miraculous ways to lengthen our lives. Part of me thinks it might be fun to rocket to Venus to celebrate my 150th birthday. The rest of me, though, would rather stay home and have my family and friends surprise me with a birthday cake (homemade, from scratch) and a sing-along around the piano— Jerome Kern, Cole Porter, George Gershwin . . .

Venus? Not me. Let's send all the rappers there instead.

Queen of the Senior Prom

My mother, who had always done everything quickly, died very efficiently of a sudden heart attack; and my devastated father succumbed to a stroke a few months later. If they had lived, I swore, I would not have put them into a long-term care facility; I would have gladly taken care of them myself at home. Of course, that was easy to say, not having been put to the test.

However, a short time later, Providence zapped me when my elderly widowed Aunt Gerlanda, whom I loved, developed serious heart problems. Her doctor said she could not live alone. I should have her move in with me, I thought. Then I thought again. She would be unattended all day while I was working, which was dangerous enough; and since she was an Olympic-class worrier, she would literally fret herself to death if I was late getting home. Also, selfishly, I knew I could say good-bye to vacations or even overnight trips or evening outings.

Trying to exorcise visions of my dear Uncle Al, Aunt Gerlanda's adoring husband, looking down from heaven and pointing an accusing finger at me, I passed the buck. I left the decision to her. God bless her, though I know it was the hardest thing she ever had to do in a life that was often very difficult, she said she wanted to go to a nursing home. She realized that coming to live with me would change my life radically, and she could not tolerate that. But I knew how terrified she was, on many levels, at the alternative on which she insisted.

First, though we've all met clean freaks, all the others are amateurs compared to my Aunt Gerlanda. She never simply washed a dish; she sterilized it. A speck of dust was an endangered species in her house; and hers were the only floors (including the bathroom tiles) from which one actually could eat with impunity. In fact, her floors were probably cleaner than the china in a five-star restaurant. The finest nursing home, or even the most luxurious hotel, could not match her standards. Then neither could my house; and because of her weakened condition, she would not be able to "Gerlandize" it.

An even more formidable barrier was her fear of strangers. Aunt Gerlanda was excruciatingly shy with people outside her immediate family. Born in Italy, she had come to America at the age of sixteen. Even though she soon learned English and spoke it beautifully, she was extremely self-conscious of her slight accent that was lovely to everyone's ears but hers. Because of her reserve, she was painfully uncomfortable with nonfamily members. I knew the thought of living with people she did not know, and to whom she was convinced she could never relate, petrified her. Nevertheless, her resolve never wavered as we approached her future one step at a time.

After thorough research, I found a lovely facility a few miles from my home so I could visit often. Smiling gallantly, she moved in. Of course, it was a complete change for her; but after a brief period of adjustment, I believe she was happy there; because in that nurturing environment, my Aunt Gerlanda discovered a new person. Herself. She even acquired a new name. Dubbed "Gerry" by her roommate. Gerry she was to one and all. To her great surprise (but certainly not mine), they all loved her. Everyone pleaded for her to sit at their table in the dining room; all sought her company throughout the day. Never a complainer, she also soon became the favorite of all the aides and the two wonderful young women social directors. They involved her in a whole range of unfamiliar activities. She shone and won prizes in most, including bowling. She had never bowled in her life. A genteel Italian senora, she would never have previously considered participating in such unladylike behavior.

When in her own home, she had seldom ventured out. Now she enjoyed day trips with the group and excursions to local restaurants. Whenever I went to visit, she was glad to see me but would soon say, "Go home. You're busy. You have a lot to do." I know she was being considerate, but I hoped that she was also eager to get back to her activities. At least I felt she was comfortable enough there to be able to urge me to leave, for whatever reason.

The highlight of her stay in the nursing home was a senior prom organized by the activities committee. The residents were asked to wear their best party clothes, and families were invited. When I received the invitation, I thought the whole idea was condescending, almost a mockery. I was wrong. Aunt Gerlanda, who had never been to a dance, anticipated it eagerly. And when she was elected prom queen, she was ecstatic. I still treasure the pictures I have of her in her gold paper crown, beaming as she danced with the social directors. Could this vivacious, bubbly Gerry be my shy, withdrawn Aunt Gerlanda?

Sadly, she died several months later. I truly believe that my Aunt Gerlanda enjoyed her last year of life as Gerry, first in the hearts of her newfound friends and queen of the senior prom.

Van Gogh and Me

I knew about Van Gogh's demons. That should have given me a clue that trying to paint will drive you crazy. As we all know, despite Vinny's amazing talent, he became so deranged that he lopped off an ear.

In my case, my staggering lack of artistic ability threatens to lead to even worse. It won't be pretty. My right hand is in imminent danger of meeting the same fate as the Van Gogh ear. Why? Because it won't do as it's told. When I put a brush in it, it stubbornly refuses to reproduce the gorgeous masterpieces pictured in my mind. Instead, it creates a mishmash of multicolored or monotoned undefined shapes. It's really very unfair. When Jackson Pollock does this, the results hang in the finest museums in the world. Mine end up in the wastebasket, torn into tiny bits, because I'm embarrassed to have the trash collector see them.

As for my endangered right hand, a key phrase in the preceding paragraph is "when I put a brush in it"—which is very seldom. How can I expect to learn to paint when I won't practice the craft? I had hoped the answer was to buy just about every book published on the subject. This might work if I would at least open one of them from time to time, but I never do. I apparently somehow believe that the wisdom they have to impart can be absorbed simply by osmosis. Hey, I do my bit. I pay good money for the books. I shouldn't have to actually read them and practice what they teach, should I?

Also, what about all those expensive brushes, paints, papers, and other accouterments that I buy? Who has the time to use them? I'm much too busy looking for excuses not to write, not to vacuum, not to practice the piano, not to exercise, not to learn Italian . . . all activities I swore I'd pursue faithfully once I retired. It's not that I haven't made an effort. I've also bought dozens of tomes (and tapes) on writing, housekeeping hints, piano playing, exercise, and Italian. Again, I haven't actually opened any of those books yet either or put any of the tapes into my Walkman? What's the point when I'm not walking?

Getting back to the subject of painting (see how easily I'm distracted?), my initial efforts were very promising. Two years ago, I took a course titled Watercolor without Fear. It was wonderful. Following the instructor's excellent guidance, I actually produced a fairly respectable painting of a rose that first evening. It was intoxicating! I was sure I had found a new career. Unfortunately, as it turned out, I have yet to surpass those premier efforts. In subsequent classes, I made the mistake of looking around at what my classmates were doing—and they were doing it so much better than me that despite my teacher's valiant attempts to encourage me, I became very intimidated.

But I'm not going to give up. In fact, first thing tomorrow morning, I'm going to rush right out and buy a great new book on watercolor techniques that I saw at Artists 'R Us last week . . . and while I'm there, I think I'll pick up that forty-nine dollar brush I've had my eye on.

The Movie Star and Me, or Beauty and the Geek

The year, 1940. The place, the Embassy Theater, a movie house in Waltham, Massachusetts.

Unlike the sterile, stark cubicles that serve as screening rooms today, the spacious Embassy was a fantasyland. It boasted a ceiling of twinkling stars against a midnight-blue sky; a huge screen draped in lush, red velvet; gilded, highly ornamented walls; uniformed (and cute!) ushers; and a richly carpeted, imposing lobby with a grand staircase curving upward to the balcony seats. In short, the Embassy was an enchanting oasis in a dreary former mill town that had morphed into a nondescript watch-manufacturing city.

I was twelve years old, painfully shy, self-conscious, gawky, and nearsighted. In that precontact lenses era, I was condemned to wearing glasses and enduring the "Four Eyes!" taunts of meanspirited classmates, which did not inspire confidence.

But at the Embassy, I forgot my insecurities, as I got lost in the wonderful world of the silver screen. One day in 1940, a memorable movie mesmerized me—*Rebecca,* starring Joan Fontaine and Laurence Olivier. He was handsome, wealthy, aloof. She was awkward, timid, withdrawn. She was me! Except she was lovely. But she didn't think so. Hey! Could it be that maybe I, too, was pretty behind my glasses but just didn't realize it? I have never identified so strongly with a character in a movie. And when she implausibly won the heart of the brooding Maxim de Winter

(Laurence Olivier), I was as ecstatic as if he were carrying *me* off to be his wife and the mistress of his mansion, Manderlay—which was even more magnificent than the Embassy Theater.

The only scenario that was even more incredible was that the woman on that screen would one day become my friend—we would correspond, chat on the phone, and even visit each other's homes. No way! Man would walk on the moon before that happened!

Well, of course, man did eventually walk on the moon; and, equally miraculously, the glamorous Joan Fontaine of Hollywood, California, did meet and befriend the shrinking violet from Waltham, Massachusetts. Both events occurred decades after that day in 1940 when *Rebecca* captured my soul and took up permanent residence there as my favorite movie of all time. Surprisingly, it is the *least* loved work of its beautiful star, even though it had won her an Oscar nomination.

I learned of Joan's aversion to *Rebecca* when I first met her in 1975. After years of slaving as Susie Steno in a series of companies, I had landed my dream job as operations manager of the Chateau de Ville, a chain of five theaters in New England, where I had the privilege of working with many of the idols of my youth—including the fabled Joan Fontaine, who had come to star in our production of *Cactus Flower*. What's more, I even got paid!

The Chateau's shows played each of our five theaters for a month, and my responsibilities included overseeing housing for the casts in each location—Spartan furnished apartments for supporting players and more luxurious digs for our stars. For the first leg of Joan's *Cactus Flower* tour with us, I had found a lovely apartment for her on Boston's Beacon Hill, overlooking the Charles River.

As soon as she was settled there, I was dispatched to pick her up and drive her to Connecticut, *Cactus Flower*'s next venue, so she could inspect some housing choices I had lined up for her there. I hadn't yet met her and was both excited and extremely nervous. I promised myself I wouldn't gush, but when she opened the door, I did just that.

"It's such a pleasure to meet you, Miss Fontaine! I absolutely loved *Rebecca!*"

I expected a "Thank you!" or at least a smile. Instead, my compliment was greeted with a frown and disconcerting silence. Huh? What was that about? I feared I was going to have to carry on a one-sided dialogue all the way to Connecticut and back. Fortunately, however, as we started down the highway, she began to relax, and conversation became very easy. She was witty, friendly, and warm. Soon I felt comfortable enough to ask her who had been her favorite leading man.

"Charles Boyer," she responded immediately. "He was a true gentleman. Working with him was a joy."

"And dare I ask who was your least favorite costar?"

Again, not a moment's hesitation. "Laurence Olivier," she replied emphatically.

Aha! A clue as to her reaction to my mention of *Rebecca.*

"The first four-letter words I ever heard were from the mouth of that man!" she added. Though the curses were not directed at her, his general surliness definitely was. Displeased because Vivien Leigh, his fiancée at the time, had not been chosen for the costarring role, he made his resentment of Joan obvious and even belittled her brand new husband, Brian Aherne, which had a devastating effect on the impressionable twenty-two-year-old bride. How then, I asked, could her and Laurence's onscreen tenderness have been so convincing?

"It's called acting, Darling," she laughed.

That day trip to Connecticut was the start of a remarkable friendship, which was cemented in the months that followed by my admiration and respect for Joan's strong work ethic and professionalism during the run of *Cactus Flower,* and later the Chateau de Ville's production of *Forty Carats* in which she also starred. Not once did she pull rank or indulge in any of the tantrums thrown by some of our other stars, despite personal difficulties that were plaguing her.

Joan was then living in a gorgeous Manhattan townhouse to which she subsequently invited me several times. She was a charming, generous, considerate hostess and incredibly unpretentious. She never fussed with hair, makeup, or clothes, yet she always looked lovely. On a rainy night when we were going to the theatre, she insisted I stay under her building's canopy while she stepped out in the downpour, sans umbrella, to hail a cab.

"I don't want you to get wet, Dear," she said when I protested.

One evening, during one of my stays, Joan apologized that she had another engagement she couldn't break, so she called a friend to escort me to the opera. On a different occasion, another of her friends took me to dinner and a Broadway show. I sure do miss that great Dial-A-Date service.

But it wasn't just the nights on the town that I enjoyed. My fondest memories of my visits include a quiet evening munching sandwiches in her cozy library where we gossiped and laughed until after midnight . . . an impromptu brunch of silver gin fizzes and eggs Benedict, whipped up by my hostess on the spur of the moment after she had urged me to cancel my early plane home and take a later flight . . . an evening when a friend dropped by and, for some reason, we all adopted the personas and Cockney accents of the servants in *Upstairs, Downstairs*, a popular British PBS show at the time. Joan was Mrs. Bridges, the cook; her friend was Hudson, the butler; and I didn't even have to change my name to be Rose, the upstairs maid. It was hilarious. No, really. Well, maybe you had to be there. I'm glad I was.

My invitations to Joan's home included a couple of Thanksgiving weekends. A Cordon Bleu graduate, she always personally prepared the elaborate holiday feast for about a dozen guests. The first time I tried to help, she frustratingly endured my bumbling efforts for five minutes before banishing me to my room to write place cards instead. Since that day, she has never let me live down my lack of culinary skills, though she did bravely accept an invitation to my home one evening when she was visiting Boston on business—and she actually ate the dinner I cooked.

Not only is Joan an exceptional chef, she's also a licensed interior decorator, a prize fisherwoman, a hot air balloonist, and a hole-in-one golfer.

"When you've had as many husbands as I've had, Love," says she, "you acquire a lot of their hobbies."

Married and divorced four times, she reflects, "If I knew when I was younger what I know now, I would have had dogs instead of husbands. They're much more faithful."

Today, she and four loyal canines, large and small, share a lovely home overlooking the Pacific in Carmel, California, where she's enjoying still another hobby—horticulture. When I visited her there one September, her sprawling garden was ablaze with a staggering array of multicolored roses, all planted and tended to by Joan herself. And it wasn't unusual to see her wielding a wrench to fix a balky faucet or disassembling an answering machine that had apparently gone on strike.

Yes, this lovely lady has a multitude of talents and admirable attributes, not the least of which is her delightful, sometimes wicked sense of humor that has endured through many adversities. As she revealed in her autobiography, *No Bed of Roses*, life has often been unkind to her, but she has never let it defeat her. A survivor, she manages to find humor in all but the direst situations. She loves to laugh. So do I. I think this has been one of our strongest bonds.

Every so often, it strikes me that this woman I am talking with or writing to is Joan Fontaine! Movie star! But most of the time, I completely forget all that, and she is simply Joan, my treasured friend.

Don't Mess with Mother Nature

Mother Nature—such a lovely appellation. It evokes images of a benevolent, nurturing caretaker. One who spends hours over a stove preparing homemade chicken soup to cure all your ills, who protects you from all danger, physical or emotional, and all monsters, real or imaginary. One who would never let you down.

Don't you believe it. Mother Nature can morph into a sneaky, evil, conniving witch in an instant. Get sucked into the goody-goody myth perpetuated by her public relations staff and let your guard down for just a moment, and she'll turn on you mercilessly.

I know because it happened to me yesterday.

I had a 1:00 P.M. doctor's appointment at a hospital a half-hour drive from my home. The weatherman predicted snow to begin from early to mid afternoon. Should I cancel? Nah. I'd be back home before any significant accumulation. It was only early December, after all. Not even officially winter yet. I got in my car around 12:15 and briefly wondered if I should go back in the house and grab a pair of boots, just in case. Again, nah. The snow hadn't started yet, and I'd be back in less than two hours.

Hah!

The first flakes began falling as I pulled into the hospital's parking garage. Hmmm . . . They were coming at a pretty fast clip. I was getting nervous. I parked and called my doctor's office on my cell phone.

"I'm here," I told the secretary, "but I think I'm just going to turn around and go home. I'm worried about the snow."

"Don't do that," she said. "He's ready for you, and it will take only a few minutes."

She did not lie. In twenty minutes, I was out of there—and into a huge mess. During those twenty minutes, a mass exodus of the hospital had begun. It took half an hour to exit the garage and maneuver the fifty-yard driveway to the street, due to massive gridlock.

In another hour, I traveled a mile and a half to Route 95, a major highway I should have reached in less than five minutes. I merged into one of the four lanes that were creeping along at under five miles an hour beneath an overhead lighted sign flashing the warning, "WINTER ADVISORY, REDUCE SPEED." Someone in the Highway Department either was completely out of touch with reality or had a cruel sense of humor.

I took several deep breaths and resigned myself to the fact that I wouldn't be seeing home any time soon. I turned on the radio and tried to relax. It worked. Until I glanced at my gas gauge and saw I had less than a quarter of a tank left. Well, at the rate of speed I was traveling, I couldn't be guzzling much fuel.

My next goal was to reach another major artery, Route 93, about eight miles away. I got there two hours later and breathed a sigh of relief. I was sure conditions on 93 would be much better.

They were worse—and went downhill with every agonizingly slow mile as a new problem developed. My windshield iced up, despite the blast of heat from my defroster. The wipers, also coated in ice, were completely ineffective. I had zero visibility. I cautiously pulled over to the side of the highway to scrape my windshield and wipers. I wasn't alone. Several other drivers had stopped to do the same thing. By the time I got back into the car, a new coat of ice had formed, and I could see nothing as I eased back onto the highway seriously believing I would die at any moment. Either I was going to smash into a car I couldn't see or another visually impaired driver was going to skid into mine. I was terrified and my gas gauge needle was now hovering close to the "Empty" mark.

I was out of options. I had to leave the highway at the next exit ramp. At least I hoped it was an exit ramp. I couldn't really tell.

Off the highway, conditions were even worse. The street was unplowed, and without taillights of other cars to guide me, and my windshield still iced, I wasn't at all sure I was even still on a road.

They say there are no atheists in foxholes; and I was certain there were also none on the highways and byways that night. I do know that God eventually guided me to a gas station. There was no way I could have reached it on my own. But once there, he deserted me. In his defense, I'm sure he was very busy answering emergency calls for help from thousands of other panicked motorists; but he could have stuck by me a few more seconds to be sure I could open the door to my gas tank. He didn't, and I couldn't. It was frozen solid under a sheet of ice. I chipped and scraped and cursed. Hey, God had left, so he wouldn't know. I finally gave up and plowed knee deep through the snow (no boots, remember?) to the gas station's convenience store to buy some deicer. I temporarily forgot how terrified I had been trying to drive since trying to walk evoked other fears—I was still recovering from recent knee surgery after I broke my patella in a fall, and I was petrified of falling again. The young clerk took pity on me and came out to help. He also chipped and scraped. And scratched, I'm sure; but at that point, I didn't care. Finally, he pried the gas tank door open. Hallelujah! I was able to fill the tank.

I cautiously rejoined the creeping traffic, but for only thirty yards or so before my windshield and wipers iced up again. I pulled into a Dunkin' Donuts parking lot and actually cried. I knew I would never make it another fifteen miles to my home. Though I've always claimed I'd rather die than impose on anyone, when death became a distinct probability instead of a hypothetical concept, I phoned my friend Mike who lived less than a mile away. He was not surprised at my predicament. His wife had just arrived home after twenty miles—and six hours!—of similar highway horror. He told me to sit tight, and he would come to rescue me. He eventually arrived, and we set out for his house.

"Am I on the road?" he kept asking me. "I can't see the road!"

Neither could I. Miraculously, we made it to his home without damage to life or limb, or Mike's car.

The next day the streets were plowed down to the pavement, and the sun shone brightly. Mother Nature was on her best behavior again. But I don't trust her for a second. I'm not leaving home again until May.

I hope I don't run out of milk—or, more important, Scotch.

The Travel Bug Will Bite You if You Don't Watch Out

I was thirty years old when I took my first trip to Europe, and I did so with reluctance and misgivings.

I had never had any desire whatsoever to roam. I'm not sure why. Fear wasn't stopping me. The word "terrorist" wasn't yet part of the travel vocabulary in that innocent age, and the thought of flying intrigued rather than intimidated me. But it didn't tempt me enough to want to leave the familiar, comfortable confines of home, so I kept turning down invitations to join friends with wanderlust—until I had a run-in with an impossible boss whose demands were becoming increasingly unreasonable.

As his overworked and underpaid secretary, I never took coffee or lunch breaks, and I always toiled way past the closing bell (yes, I actually toiled, and yes, we actually had a bell), as well as on several weekends and holidays—all without extra compensation. I even typed his wife's weekly nursery-school-association newsletters on my lunch hours.

One day, goaded by his command to draw a school bus on one of said newsletters (despite my protests that I had no artistic ability), I perversely told him I'd like to take an extra two weeks' vacation, without pay, that year to travel to Europe with my friend Sally who had been begging me to accompany her. My request was not unusual. Many others in the company, which had several overseas divisions, did this regularly. His immediate response (which I, of course, had anticipated) was,

"Absolutely not. I can't spare you."

"I understand," I nodded, and then went directly to my cubicle and dialed Sally.

"Make the reservations," I said.

Thus began my long love affair with travel. I owe that boss big time. I forced myself to take my first trip to spite him, but I ended up loving every minute of it and making up for lost time since then by trekking to far-off lands whenever I had the chance.

It's incredible how travel has changed since my first trip. Interminable, noisy, propeller-powered flights have been replaced by swift, quiet jets—with movies and music to make the time seem even shorter. Lightweight suitcases (with wheels!) have made our rigid, hefty luggage obsolete. Comfortable clothing has superseded the dresses, high-heels, nylon stockings—and girdles—which were *de rigueur* back then (at least for females). In one way, I miss the former formality that lent a touch of glamour to travel. However, I do *not* miss being pained, pinched, and constricted from head to toe—not only during a transatlantic flight, but also after arrival while seeing the sights.

And I'm deliriously happy that those comfortable clothes are also carefree, thanks to fabric blends that resist creasing, even when crushed into a suitcase, and dry wrinkle-free a couple of hours after being dunked in a bathroom sink. No more need to tote cumbersome electric current converters for those small, but heavy, travel irons we lugged and had to spend precious minutes using before we were able to go out and see the wonders of Paris . . . the grandeur of Rome . . . the cute surfer dudes on Waikiki . . .

Neither do I miss having to pack (and keep track of) a couple of dozen rolls of film and worrying about having my pictures destroyed by the security X-rays at airports. Today, an X-ray-proof, miniscule memory card in my tiny digital camera captures hundreds of images. What's more, I can see the results immediately on the camera's LCD screen and reshoot if an unexpected snag has sabotaged my first effort. This is so much better than being kept in suspense until I get home and have film developed only to find a close-up of my camera strap instead of a shot of the Eiffel Tower, the corner of a *carabiniere's* wind-blown cape instead of that great shot I thought I had of the Pope, or my tour leader's alpine hat obscuring the Matterhorn.

Another boon to modern travel is the ATM, which eliminates the necessity of carrying large amounts of currency. Pickpockets aren't too happy about this, but you didn't travel all that way to enrich their lives, did you?

Not all the changes are for the better, however. Take, for example, cell phones, laptops, Blackberries, and other communication devices. At first, we might think they're a boon because no matter how far we roam, they keep us in touch with our families, friends, and business associates—which, come to think of it, is exactly why they're a terrible idea. When you're on vacation, do you really want to hear that your son flunked his finals (right after your $40,000 check for that year's tuition cleared), your daughter is thinking of moving in with that loser she's been dating, the nursing home is threatening to expel your grandfather because he was streaking through the halls again, or that your company is downsizing and your job is on the line? It was better before when the only way anyone from home could reach you was via a prohibitively expensive transoceanic phone call that was so static-ridden you couldn't understand a word.

There are exceptions, of course. My friend Jean recently went to Venice, a magical place her incapacitated grandmother had always dreamed of visiting some day. Jean couldn't help her fulfill that fantasy, so she did the next best thing. While gliding along the Grand Canal in a gondola, she slipped her cell phone from her bag, dialed her grandmother, and asked the gondolier to serenade her. He happily obliged, and Granny was thrilled.

"Even Pavarotti never sang 'O Sole Mio' as beautifully," she blubbered. "It's almost as good as being there!"

Almost isn't good enough for me. I still haven't recovered from my decades-old bite of the travel bug. In fact, if it weren't for financial concerns, I'd hop on the next jet to almost anywhere. Well, maybe hopping is out (bad knees), but I'd clamber aboard somehow.

I'll be back in Capri tomorrow if I win the lottery tonight.

First, I have to buy a ticket.

The Attack of
the Vengeful Veggies

Help! I'm being terrorized by a giant zucchini—and a green pepper, a bag of baby carrots, and a head of wilted romaine lettuce.

Well, maybe "terrorized" is a bit strong; but these assorted veggies are certainly seriously intimidating me. Every time I open my refrigerator door, they say (I swear they can talk),

"Eat me! Throw away that cookie! You don't need that jelly doughnut! Eat *me!* Don't let me rot!"

The irony of the situation is that they couldn't have any power over me at all if I hadn't brought them home from the supermarket and given them haven in my fridge in the first place. You'd think I would have learned my lesson by now. But I haven't. I make the same mistake every time I go grocery shopping. Last week my tormenters were two artichokes, some string beans, spinach, and a bunch of beets, all of which I eventually fed to my garbage disposal.

Why do I keep buying things I probably won't eat? Because they're good for me, and I know I *should* eat them. Instead, however, I usually plop a big greasy hamburger on the grill; but I do put ketchup on it and eat chips with it—don't they count as two veggies? Or I'll dig into a heaping plate of pasta but with tomato sauce and some fresh chopped basil (there you go—something green!) so it can't be all that bad. Or if I'm feeling virtuous, I'll eat chicken. Everyone knows that chicken is certainly healthier than the juicy, marbled sirloin steak I'd rather have. Okay, okay—so I prefer the dark meat thighs and drumsticks instead of the leaner white meat breasts; and yes, I do fry them but in virgin olive oil, which is good for LDL cholesterol, isn't it?

I know I'm just rationalizing my poor choices.

It isn't that I dislike vegetables. I eat (and enjoy) them when others prepare them. But when I have to do it myself, it's just too much work. All that washing, peeling, dicing, slicing, chopping, mashing. Not to mention the boiling, braising, roasting, steaming, stewing—followed by the scouring and washing of all the pans, knives, choppers, mashers. Seriously, far fewer utensils are involved in broiling or frying a piece of meat or boiling a pot of water for pasta. And fewer still for fast food takeout.

Despite that, starting tomorrow I'm going to prepare meals that are more nutritious. Sure I am. But I tell myself that every day, and it hasn't happened yet. It's easy to make that vow right after I've polished off a large baguette slathered with mayonnaise and overstuffed with roast beef, ham, salami, and three kinds of cheese and garnished with bacon bits (okay, slabs).

Sometimes I actually remember my promise the next morning. Those are the days I raid the vegetable bins at the supermarket. Unfortunately, I have to pass Pizzeria Uno on the way home; but I don't—pass it, that is. All that grocery shopping makes me hungry, so I decide to go in and have a light lunch—just one slice of pizza. I'll bring the rest home and freeze it to serve to my Scrabble group on Sunday. Inevitably, one slice leads to another, and I polish off the whole thing—so I buy another one for my company on Sunday. Well, I have to offer them something. Of course, I do have all that produce in my crispers, but I don't think a vegetable medley will cut it with this group. In addition to the pizza, I know they'll be expecting munchies like Tostitos and salsa, cheese and crackers, chips and dip, nuts and pretzels. Is it my fault that they have such poor eating habits?

As for me, I really am going to make an effort to improve my diet—starting right now with a nice glass of wine. (Hey, it's grape juice, after all.)

The Good Old Days–Not!
(Memoirs of a Former Secretary)

Remember the offices of yesterday—when the woman who did ten times the work of the boss (male, of course) for one-tenth the pay wasn't an executive assistant? Back then, she was called a secretary. She was also called a girl, as in, "Let's set a meeting date. . . . I'll have my girl call your girl."

Not only did we "girls" get no respect. We also had no word processing. What we had was the typewriter. For young people who may never have seen one of these ancient contraptions (and for former bosses who wouldn't demean themselves by getting within spitting distance of one), a description follows:

A typewriter was a single-unit machine with a keyboard similar to that of a computer, but without the function keys. No monitors. No printers. Instead, the typewriter incorporated a roller device above the keyboard. The typist would wind paper into the roller, and as she (typists were never "he") struck the keys, she activated individual levers, one for each letter and symbol, which would spring up and transfer the corresponding character to the paper in the roller. This was pre-electric machines. I'm talking manual here—clunkers with keys that one had to **POUND** to activate. We girls practiced for years in order to increase finger agility and speed. But when we achieved those goals, we were stymied, because if we typed too fast, the levers would all pile up on each other, like mad dogs in heat, and would jam.

The characters were transferred to the paper through the

magic of a typewriter ribbon—a heavily inked, narrow band of fabric on a spool. We had to wind this ribbon through an intricate pathway of metal guides and then attach it to a take-up spool on the opposite end of the machine. In the process of installing a new ribbon, we usually managed to transfer most of the ink that was originally on the ribbon to our hands and clothes. Consequently, after we typed a few pages, the print on the paper would become so faint, we would have to install a new ribbon.

We also had no copying machines in the good old days. In order to make copies of anything we typed, we used carbon paper. Remember that? It was smooth on one side, heavily inked on the other. We would make multidecker paper "sandwiches"—the original on top, backed up by tissue-thin sheets called onionskin, one for each copy needed, with sheets of carbon paper interspersed between the onionskins. When a typewriter key was struck, in addition to leaving its mark on the original, it would also transfer ink from the carbon sheets to the onionskins. Unfortunately, the impression would be fainter on each succeeding copy. By the time the key hit copy number five or six, you could barely tell it had been there. This meant, of course, that when we needed more copies, we would have to retype an original with yet another carbon stack. As if once wasn't bad enough. If we were unfortunate enough to make a mistake, we had no delete key to fix it. We had to erase each copy separately, inserting slips of paper between each carbon and onionskin to prevent smudging as we erased the top sheets. We would then erase each copy separately and remove the slips of paper before we resumed typing—if we remembered, that is.

No copying machines also meant that when we were sending someone an enclosure—an article from a newspaper, a letter received from someone else, the company's P&L statement—if we needed to keep a copy, we had to type the whole damn thing! And what if we wanted to send copies of the enclosures to anyone else? See "carbon paper" above.

Almost forgot (or I tried to repress the memory): We actually did have other means of making multiple copies of documents for wider distribution. One was the Ditto machine. A fiendish invention that distributed indelible purple ink on a master that we typed—as well as on our clothes, hands, feet, and, by some mysterious process, even unexposed body parts. We then affixed this master to a cylinder on the Ditto machine and turned it with a crank to run off copies.

The mimeograph machine was another diabolic duplicating device. If we didn't want to get purple ink all over ourselves, instead of using a ditto master, we typed a mimeograph stencil. This was a blue sheet over a stiff backing on which we typed without a typewriter ribbon so that the keys cut through the stencil. If we made a mistake, we coated it with a special white glop, waited for it to dry, and then tried to cut the correct symbols through the glop. Good luck. When the typing and glopping were finished, we wrapped the stencil around the black-ink coated drum of the mimeograph machine and cranked out the required copies. The big advantage of this method was no purple-stained clothes and body parts. We did, however, wind up with black-stained clothes and body parts.

Of course, none of these inconveniences affected the boss. He was oblivious to them all. He never had to deal with them. He just lounged in his spacious, windowed office and dictated or scrawled his communications. Susie Secretary, at her cramped desk in the servants' quarters, did the rest.

In addition, she also brewed and served his coffee, and made reservations for his expense-paid leisurely lunches at costly cafés. And while the boss was enjoying his martinis and oysters Rockefeller, Susie was at her desk, trying to eat a brown-bag peanut butter sandwich while typing Mrs. Boss's club meeting's minutes.

Surprisingly, though Susie was often a bright woman and maybe even had as much, or maybe more, education than her boss, she was so brainwashed that it never occurred to her that something was wrong with this picture. She was happy she had a job. Furthermore, she got a whole week off—with pay! And after five years, she could look forward to *two* weeks with pay. Boy, those were the good old days.

NOT!

I'm Sorry . . . Do I Know You?

So you can't remember names, and you think that's a problem. Tough toenails (as I used to say before I dumped my old crowd and joined a more sophisticated circle).

But back to your so-called dilemma. You get no sympathy from me because I have a much worse problem: Though I have little difficulty recalling names, I have absolutely no memory for faces. And I can't even blame my aging brain. This affliction has plagued me all my life.

That's not so terrible, you say. Really? Look at it this way. What's the good of having lots of names on the tip of your tongue if you don't know when to spit them out? On the other hand, if you remember faces but not names, you have it made. When you're at a party or walking down the street and you bump into someone you've met, you can smile brightly and say, "Hey! Good to see ya!" or "How absolutely delightful to have encountered you!" depending on your own sophistication level.

Me, I walk right by without a flicker of recognition, leaving the other person assuming I'm an obnoxious snob. It's painfully embarrassing, especially if I had just had breakfast with that person a couple of hours before . . . or if he's the man who had filled in as a substitute at bridge the previous week . . . or if she's the woman to whom I had given a card last May that said, "To My Wonderful Mother."

Okay, so that last example is a slight exaggeration. Actually, I do recognize close friends and relatives. However, if I see most other people outside of the environments with which I associate them, they might as well be total strangers. For example, last December when I was clearing snow from my car in front of my house, a man drove up, got out of his car, and offered to help. I thought it was the guy who had just moved out of the condo next to mine. Wrong. It was my financial adviser whom I have visited regularly for the past fifteen years. He had come by to drop off a Christmas present. But because he was wearing a ski parka instead of a business suit and he wasn't behind his desk, I didn't recognize him.

Most people cannot identify with such experiences. One friend is particularly skeptical. That's because she remembers everyone she ever met since she was two years old, even if she hasn't seen them in fifty years and they've had three facelifts in the interim. Then she rubs it in by saying something like, "You'd have known her, too—she has the same look around the eyes as she had in the second grade."

Yeah, right. Like I'd remember how someone's eyes had looked like this morning, never mind decades ago.

I not only can't convince this particular friend that I'm not lying, I've come close to losing other newer friends whose feelings are hurt to think they apparently made so little impression on me that I don't even recognize them.

If I hear later that I've inadvertently snubbed someone, I of course try to explain. Fortunately, I now have ammunition to back up my apology. I Googled the Internet and found dozens of Web sites about my handicap. It seems I have an actual scientific malady called prosopagnosia, or facial blindness, a condition caused by faulty cranial wiring, probably a second cousin to dyslexia, that causes us to forget facial features. Until research proved they are often brighter than average, people with dyslexia were thought to be stupid. I'd like to think that this is also true of those of us with prosopagnosia.

But I won't flaunt my superior intelligence if you promise not to be angry if I don't speak to you the next time I see you.

Be My Guest

"You're staying with us while you're in town. No way are you going to a hotel when we have an empty guest room just going to waste."

"It's been so long since we've seen you. Surely you can get away for at least a week?"

"Please come for a visit! It will be fun!"

You've had similar invitations, I'm sure. And if you've accepted them, like me, you've had a delightful time—or not.

I have enjoyed some of the best getaways of my life visiting friends whose five-star hospitality included luxurious accommodations and unlimited pampering and coddling. Annie didn't have it as good at Daddy Warbucks' digs.

However, some other experiences—not so great.

A while back I visited friends in Florida who ensconced me in their "guest room"—a tiny den/office with a foldaway bed that almost engulfed the entire room when opened. The only lamp was on top of a high chest wedged next to the bed. In order to turn off the lamp, I had to stand up on the bed, which resulted in the diabolical contraption folding up and trapping my legs in a viselike grip. When I finally extricated myself and managed to lie down, an iron bar under the thin mattress made sleep impossible. I spent the night mentally composing a letter to Congress demanding they enact a law requiring people to try to sleep in their own guest rooms before foisting them on unsuspecting visitors.

I once accepted a summer weekend invitation from a friend in a remote area of Maine. She didn't tell me until after I arrived, on the hottest day of the year, that the area had no electricity, which meant no air conditioning, no refrigeration, no TV, no reading in bed . . . and no way to find the bathroom at 3:00 A.M. without risking falling down the stairs, stubbing my toes on furniture in my path, or tripping over Fran. No, not my hostess—her pet goat, who had somehow managed to push open the back door and enter the house.

But that was preferable to the night I stayed with another friend in Manhattan who shared her tiny sixth-floor walk-up with millions of dust mites (who apparently hadn't been disturbed in months) and seven cats with weak bladders (and no litter box). I concentrated on not inhaling all night while I invented an "emergency" that would require me to leave at dawn.

As unpleasant as those (and several other unfortunate sojourns) were, the prize for my worst guest experience goes to what I will always remember as my California catastrophe:

Many years ago, when I was planning a business trip to the West Coast, I phoned Ellen, a former coworker who had moved to San Francisco. I asked if she could meet me for lunch or dinner on one of the two days I'd be there so we could catch up on each other's lives.

"I'm staying at the Marriott at Fishermen's Wharf," I told her.

"No, you're not!" ordered Ellen. "You're staying with us."

"Us?" I asked.

"Paul and me," she said. "We have a great house with a swimming pool, just a few miles out of town.

"Paul? Not the Paul you used to date back here in Boston?"

"That's right. Remember? He moved to California a few years ago?"

I had never met Paul, but I did recall her hysterical meltdown when he left town.

"Well," Ellen continued. "When he heard I was coming west, he absolutely insisted I move in with him."

News to me. Gossip had it that the reason Paul had moved

three thousand miles away was to escape from Ellen. Apparently, absence had made his heart grow fonder. Good for her.

"That's great, Ellen," I said, "but I really have to be in the city for my appointments, and . . ."

"No problem," she interrupted. "You can borrow my car. It's settled. What time does your flight get in? I'll pick you up."

I finally reluctantly agreed.

Stupid!

Ellen collected me at the airport, and we drove a few miles east to a pleasant suburb with modest houses on postage-stamp-sized lots. Paul wasn't home, but Ellen assured me he was really looking forward to my visit. Very much the grand dame of the domain, she proudly gave me a tour of the house and its miniscule pool that comprised the entire backyard.

She then proceeded to cook dinner.

"Your stomach is still on East Coast time; you must be starving," she said. "Paul will be home by six."

At eight, we were still waiting for Paul, while the chicken grew cold, the gravy congealed, the salad wilted, and the soufflé collapsed. She served it all anyway, and I made a valiant effort to down a few mouthfuls.

Paul staggered in at ten. That was the good news. The bad news was that he wasn't alone. With him was a woman with whom he had apparently been partying. Ellen was furious. Paul and the girl friend turned on the stereo and started drunkenly dancing and nuzzling, paying no attention whatsoever to Ellen's verbal barrage.

"I can't believe you'd do this to me when you knew we were having a guest!" she shrieked.

I motioned her out of the room.

"I shouldn't be here," I told her. "Please call a taxi for me."

"Absolutely not!" she said, insisting that when Paul sobered up, he'd be very upset if I left.

"It's that bitch!" she said. "She's always pulling something like this—getting him drunk and taking advantage of him!"

Always? This happened a lot?

"Ellen, I *really* want to leave," I pleaded.

Not possible, she said. The cabs did not operate late at night, and she couldn't drive me back to the city because "the bitch's" car was parked behind hers. My only escape was to the guest room.

Ellen led me to it and put on her hostess face again.

"It's a waterbed," she said, indicating a monstrous blob that dominated the room. "You'll love it."

Wrong. She had forgotten to turn on the bed's heater; and despite lying on top of, instead of under, the bed quilt, I felt as though I were on an ice floe in the North Atlantic. Whenever I moved to curl up into a tighter ball to expose the least body surface possible to the chill, the mattress undulated wildly, threatening to pitch me to the floor. I was seasick. My teeth were chattering. I couldn't sleep. And not just because of the discomfort. Also keeping me awake was a ferocious argument that started downstairs and then continued upstairs, after "the bitch" had left. I heard language, from both Ellen and Paul, that would be bleeped in a XXX-rated movie.

Ellen was still playing the wronged, outraged mate while Paul thundered that she had no business telling him what to do—and, for that matter, no right to be living in his house. He reminded her that she had showed up uninvited one day and had been foiling his attempts to evict her ever since. So much for the romantic fairytale she had spun for me.

The argument grew more violent. I heard scuffling. I heard blows. I heard objects being flung. I remembered seeing a shotgun in a case in the den. Was it loaded? Would one of them go for it? Would a bullet come through the wall and pierce the waterbed, flooding the room with an icy torrent? Even if I knew how to swim, I'd succumb to hypothermia.

What in God's name was I doing here? Oh, how I wished I were at the Marriott!

The next morning, Paul apologized for making me feel

"uncomfortable" (the understatement of the century) as Ellen tried to hand me her car keys so I could drive to my appointment. That, of course, meant I'd have to drive back. Another night in Madhouse Manor? No way. I dialed 411 for the number of the local cab company and made my escape.

Despite the good manners my mother had instilled in me, I simply could not write a "thank you so much for your hospitality" note.

I never heard from Ellen again.

I've learned my lesson. From now on, before I accept an overnight invitation, I shall demand references from former guests, a notarized list of amenities that will be provided, affidavits from OSHA and the local health and police departments that the environment is safe and clean, plus—in cases where there will be more than one host—a sworn statement from a clergyman attesting that they have a tender, loving relationship.

Otherwise, I'm going to the Marriott.

The Secret in the Freezer
(And Other Scandals)

Last night I jolted awake from a sound sleep, panicked that I might suffer a sudden heart attack or speech-robbing stroke before daylight. A distressing concern any time, of course, but especially last night. Why? Because of what relatives or friends might find in my freezer after I was taken away.

No, I hadn't murdered and dismembered my nosy neighbor and hidden her body parts there (not that I haven't been tempted at times). Nor were any packages of mystery meat or other unidentified fossilized foods tucked back in the corners as testimony of my sloppy housekeeping. And neither was I hiding a secret stash of vodka.

So what was I afraid they'd find? A shoe stuffed with a plastic bag of ice and sheathed in two grocery bags.

I can hear them now:

"I knew she was losing it, but this is ridiculous!"

"Was she planning to defrost it for dinner?"

"Maybe someone told her to cool her heels and she took it literally."

"Tsk! Tsk! Poor Rosie."

Actually, I had a perfectly logical reason for filing footwear in the freezer; but if I were struck dead or speechless, I'd never be able to explain that I was simply implementing a tip I had read the day before about how to stretch a too-tight shoe (i.e., put some water in a plastic bag, seal it, stuff the bag into the shoe, and put it in the freezer overnight). As the water in the bag freezes and expands, it will enlarge the shoe.

See. Not crazy after all. Brilliant, actually, because it worked.

And that got me thinking about other stuff I'd hate to have anyone discover if I'm suddenly whisked away:

My junk drawer in my kitchen, for instance, which is crammed with, well, junk.

"What in heaven's name is this rusty thing-a-ma-jig?" they'd ponder. (I don't know either. I've had it for years and never figured out what it was, but I didn't want to throw it out because I might need it some day.)

"A meat thermometer—yeah, like she ever cooked a roast."

"Look, a garlic press. Just last week she told me she wanted one for her birthday. She obviously didn't realize she already had one."

Not to mention the broken corkscrew . . . the turkey baster ("Roast a turkey? Rosie? Right.") . . . the flashlight with the corroded batteries . . . the hammer with the loose handle . . .

So that's where those are! I've been looking for them for years.

The kitchen isn't the only room in the house I'd be embarrassed to have submitted to postmortem scrutiny. A visit to the dining room would soon expose the shameful fact that I haven't polished my silverware in eons. (Trust me. I'm sure there are eating utensils somewhere under all that tarnish.)

In the living room, they would wonder anew why I still have a piano and all those music books.

"She was delusional—kept saying she was going to start practicing and playing again; but, to be fair, she never specified in which lifetime."

The bedroom would reveal a further shocker. No, not a drawer full of sex toys, but a closet full of should-be castoffs.

"Ninety percent of this stuff should have gone to Goodwill— fifty years ago! What was she saving it all for?"

"She was right when she used to say she had nothing to wear— nothing here is fit to wear, that's for sure!"

"And size 8 jeans! Probably the last time she was able to get into these was when she was twelve!"

Wrong. When I was twelve, girls didn't wear jeans. Just ladylike dresses and skirts. In fact, I *never* wore the size 8 jeans. I bought them as an incentive ten years ago when I was starting a new diet. I'm still waiting to squeeze into them, which might happen after I master the piano.

"You think the stuff in the closet is bad? Take a look at her costume jewelry collection. . . . 'Costume' is right—Halloween is the only time I'd wear it—and then only if I covered it with a ghost sheet!"

"Okay, who's going to look under the bed?"

"Not me. I just poked my foot there, and I swear something moved. Anything could be living there."

"Hey! Check out this linen closet. She's got frayed towels here dating back to the royal wedding—Albert and Victoria's!"

"Seven bottles of hair color! And no two are the same brand or shade. CVS must have had a sale of leftovers."

All this is bad enough but pales in comparison to what they'll say when they get to my office/den/guest room. The mere fact that this room serves three functions makes it a natural repository for a hodgepodge of "stuff" (that's the only word for it).

Hand weights and an exercise ball (all never used, by the way) . . . a pile of disorganized papers as high as Everest on the computer desk (yes, there really is a computer buried there, too—keep digging) . . . more papers strewn on the sofa bed and coffee table . . . books tumbling out of bookcases . . . a broken VCR blinking twelve o'clock . . . file cabinets jammed with unfinished projects . . . and all this on a good day, after I've tidied up. Oh yes, my cleaner-uppers will have a field day in here.

My friend Jane never has to fear similar embarrassing revelations. A minimalist to the 'nth degree, she doesn't allow even an extra postage stamp to clutter a drawer (an actual example, swear to God). In fact, Jane's home has been pristinely cleared for her take-off from this planet for more than thirty years. It's so shipshape, her survivors will have to go someplace else to find a match for the crematorium.

Today's the day for me to begin to become more Jane-like, to clean out extraneous miscellany and get organized. I started by making a detailed "to-do" list this morning. Unfortunately, I can't remember where I put it.

Maybe I should check the freezer.

The U.S. Postal Disservice

It gets worse every day. It's bad enough that I have to dial eleven digits to phone my neighbor across the hall, but at least I can still get through to her personally. Not so any more with my local post office, three miles away.

It was 4:30 P.M. I had a package to mail. I didn't know if my post office closed at 4:30 or 5:00. I dialed its number. A robotic voice referred me to an 800 number that, in turn, connected me to someone in Denver, Colorado—two thousand miles from my home. Correction: the 800 number actually did not connect me to an actual human being in Denver—not until I listened to eleven (there's that number again) menu options.

You know the drill: Starting with the usual "for English press 1, for Spanish press 2" and proceeding through six other choices, depending on whether I wanted information on mailing a letter or package (Press 1), rates (2), zip codes (3), reporting an address change or placing mail on vacation hold (4), delivery of mail to my business or residence (5), or other postal information (6). That last one sounded encouraging. I pressed 6 and was rewarded with still more choices:

"If you are calling about retail products or services, press 1; if you are calling about postal services provided by your delivery unit, press 2; if you wish to speak to a customer service representative, press 3 . . ."

I did—press 3, that is—and finally heard a live person! I told her I simply wanted to know what time my post office closed. She was very pleasant. She said she'd be happy to help. She asked for my zip code and put me on hold. I held until my question became moot. It was too late to go to the post office by now, even if it closed at five.

A few months ago, I went away on a vacation. I had requested my post office to hold my mail. After a couple of days, my neighbor called me to let me know my mail was still being delivered. I phoned my post office and spoke to the postmaster who apologized and assured me he would remind my delivery person to hold my mail. Problem solved. If the same thing happens the next time I go away, I doubt if that nice woman in Denver could help; she probably wouldn't be able to get through to my local post office either.

And now postage is going up—again . . . all of which supports my long-held theory that postal rates increase in direct proportion to the decrease in service.

If the Post Office Department is adamant about maintaining this new disservice, I suggest they add one more option to the menu: "If this system is driving you crazy and you'd like a referral to a psychiatrist, press eleventeen."

The Curse of Punctuality

Those who studied Grimm in kindergarten prep remember how the wicked fairy, miffed at not being invited to the royal christening, crashed the party to get even by laying a curse on the baby princess. Fortunately, Nasty Nellie arrived late, after the infant had already been guaranteed wealth, beauty, wisdom, and long life by the good fairies with bona fide invitations. Consequently, the worst curse old Nell could conjure up was that the princess would sleep for one hundred years. A century later, she was awakened by the kiss of a handsome prince. And since there were no in-laws left to bother him, he became a devoted husband and, of course, they lived happily ever after. So what was intended as a curse turned out to be a blessing.

In my case, it was just the opposite. Since I wasn't born into royalty, the good fairies politely declined invitations to my christening. Even wicked Nellie (yeah, she was still around) figured it would be a drag and didn't come. So not only was I deprived of wealth, wisdom, and beauty, but I was also cheated of a century-long nap. The good fairies, however, did chip in and send me, via Western Union (this was before e-mail, of course), one old, unused blessing. I still have the wire: WELCOME! MAY YOU ALWAYS BE PUNCTUAL. LOVE, THE GIRLS.

They meant well, but their blessing turned out to be a curse. From the moment that telegram arrived, I was doomed to a wasted life of endless waiting for others, since none of my friends was similarly blessed. Instead, they're all wealthy, wise, good-looking—and late. Constantly, dependably, unfailingly late. I estimate that over the last five years alone I've spent at least one thousand hours waiting for people.

I've waited on cold, windy street corners, whiling away the time watching the passing scene—until I get so upset and angry-looking that the passing scene starts watching me.

I've waited in shops until the store detective begins to wonder if I'm shoplifting very cleverly alone or waiting for my accomplices to bring the guns. To calm him, I start buying things I don't need. (Anyone want some wrinkle cream? No, wait! I do need that.)

In the summer, I've waited on hot, dusty park benches, squandering my week's grocery budget on peanuts to appease the squirrels and pigeons who have come to think of me as a mobile branch of the Salvation Army soup kitchen.

When I invite friends home for dinner, invariably the ice cubes in the wine cooler bucket melt and the soufflé collapses long before the first guest arrives.

It's even worse to make the mistake of arriving at someone else's home at the appointed hour. The last time I did this, I found my bathrobe-clad hostess, cream on her face and hair in rollers, mumbling, "Oh, we didn't expect you so early!" She then disappeared into her boudoir leaving me with the canapés to fix and the feeling that I had committed an unpardonable breach of etiquette.

Of course, you realize what a mistake it is to get to the theater on time. Some gremlin sees to it that your seats are on the aisle, and you spend the entire first act getting up to let latecomers into the row.

An even bigger blunder is to be on time to your own surprise party, which turns out to be a surprise to all the other guests when they finally show up and see you got there before them.

And woe to the bride who gets to the church on time—the most serious social gaffe possible. Let's face it. It's her last chance to play hard to get, and she blows it. Everyone assumes she's overeager. Not good.

Unfortunately, the disadvantages of punctuality aren't confined to social situations. In the hours I've spent waiting in doctors' and dentists' offices, for instance, I could have toured the world—and by tramp steamer yet.

Then there's the workplace. During my secretarial years, I found that it wasn't even worth getting to the office on time. None of the VIPs were ever there to see. And when one of the wheels finally rolled in a half-hour late and found that his own wealthy, wise, and beautiful secretary hadn't arrived yet, guess who got to type that forty-page report?

I could tell you more, but I don't have time. I'm due at a party next door in half an hour so I have to run. I don't want to be late.

Congratulations!
You're a Winner!

P. T. Barnum was right. There's a sucker born every minute. I ought to know. I'm one of them.

The thing is, I've always had a reputation for being smart. So how could I have been so stupid as to believe that letter I received last week from Honest Abe's Autos?

Abe was trying to lure me into his dealership by guaranteeing me an incredible trade-in value for my car. Because he wisely guessed that his unbelievable offer did not sound, well, believable, he enclosed an incentive—a lottery scratch card headed, "SCRATCH—MATCH—WIN! EVERY TICKET A WINNER!"

The accompanying letter promised no obligation, no pressure to consider actually trading in my car. I would simply have to pop into the dealership, and one of five possible prizes would be mine: $4,500 in cash (fat chance), a $1,000 online shopping spree (ditto), $500 in grocery coupons (which you can get with the Sunday paper and which induce you to spend big bucks for tons of stuff you don't need), $20 worth of gas (most of which, at today's prices, my car would guzzle driving to Honest Abe's), or $5 in cash (absolutely not worth the cost of the trip). However, unlike most similar promotions that require you to bring the card into the offering establishment and have a salesperson scratch it to see what you've won, this card instructed me to scratch it myself and reveal my prize. I did.

Oh, happy day! I had actually scored the $1,000 online

shopping spree! I couldn't believe it. I know it's a cliché, but I really never do win anything. I started making a mental list of the marvelous possibilities that were just a few keystrokes away, an extra memory card and battery for my digital camera to ensure I'd be able to take as many pictures as I wanted on my next trip—and, hey, maybe an airline ticket for that trip, possibly a leather coat, a new vacuum cleaner? Or maybe I'd really be impractical and blow it all on a pair of diamond earrings.

I got in my car and headed for Honest Abe's, visions of treasures dancing in my head. I'm not naïve. I knew it wouldn't be that easy. Despite the "no obligation" promise in the letter, I figured I'd have to submit to a little arm-twisting to get me to trade in my car. But those earrings were looking more dazzling with each passing mile. They'd be worth enduring a high-pressure pitch.

I presented my prizewinning lottery ticket to the salesman who approached as I entered the dealership. He asked what make and year of car I was planning to trade in.

"There's no way I can afford a new car right now," I sheepishly admitted. "I'm just here to pick up my prize."

Surprise! No coercion. No sales spiel. Apparently, his sixth sense (or maybe a quick appraisal of my bargain basement attire) confirmed that I was not a viable prospect with deep pockets and not worth any more of his valuable time.

"No problem," he smiled, opening a drawer and extracting a gift certificate. "That's it?" I asked. "No catch? I actually won a $1,000 online shopping spree?"

"That's right," he confirmed. "No catch. Congratulations!"

I couldn't wait to start shopping. I rushed home and turned on my computer. As it was booting up, I read the gift certificate. Oh, oh. I noticed one small hitch after all. I would not be able to shop on the entire World Wide Web, only on the "Rewards" address specified on the certificate. Oh, well. I was sure the site would be brimming with enough goodies to make me happy.

It wasn't.

The pickings were meager and the quality poor. They did offer a leather coat, for example; but it was "crafted" (or, rather, piecework assembled) from patchwork leather, as was the leather "luggage" (tote bags and backpacks) featured on the site. I then clicked the "Home Decor" button, thinking I could get some sheets or a new comforter; but the only product in the category was a sleazy-looking chenille throw. The fact that it was available in a variety of colors did not enhance its appeal.

I still hadn't given up. I noted a "Jewelry" tab. Hey! Maybe my diamond earrings were waiting for me there. Alas, no. Tawdry costume bling-bling were the only possibilities.

So I set my sights lower. Though all of the categories were equally sparse, maybe I could at least get a couple of new phones. Yes! There were two I could actually use! But clicking on the "Buy Now" button, brought up a window that listed "Shipping Charges." I looked at my "gift" certificate again. Sure enough, I would be responsible for separate shipping and handling fees on each item I selected. I could not use any portion of the certificate for these charges but would have to supply credit card information. For the telephones, the shipping and handling came to more than I would have to pay for new phones at my local Wal-Mart. I investigated shipping charges on other items on the site and found that some were as high as 47 percent of the supposed value of the item.

I calculated that $1,000 worth of "free" shoddy merchandise would cost me $300 to $400 in delivery fees.

As I wallowed in my disappointment, my phone rang. It was a friend calling to tell me, "Guess what? I just received a letter from Honest Abe's Autos. I won a $1,000 online shopping spree!"

Coincidence? No way. In fact, I'm sure all of the thousands of people on Honest Abe's ill-gotten mailing list won the same prize. And if even only a tiny percentage of those who visited the dealership to claim their reward were sufficiently enticed by the shiny new cars in the showroom to trade in their vehicles, Abe would make out like a bandit . . . which, come to think of it, is very appropriate.

Weather or Not

Are you a lucky weatherproof person? No, I don't mean is your skin impervious to the elements and does your hair remain frizz-free even in the tropics. What I'm asking is if your mood is unaffected by seasonal changes—your happy-go-lucky disposition undampened by sleet, subarctic blizzards, or sweltering heat and humidity.

Actually, do any such people exist? If so, I have yet to meet one. Everyone I know seems to have a definite season preference. They either relish the frigid snows of winter or flourish during summer's most blistering days.

I am ignoring those whose favorite season is spring or fall. Well, duh! Wouldn't we all wish every day to be bright and breezy, with a temperature range of sixty to eighty degrees? Actually, maybe not. A reasonably rational friend who had lived in Hawaii for more than a year claimed he became bored with perfect weather. He loved it for the first couple of months, he said, but eventually when he looked out the window in the morning, he'd groan, "Oh, no! Another #$%& beautiful day!"

Of course to those of us who live in New England, the spring/fall issue is moot. We rarely get to experience either. We might retire one night in early March, nursing our aches from shoveling the front walk for the third time that day, and awake to the birds singing and the weather gal forecasting temperatures in the nineties by noon. Then one sweltering humid night in mid September, we could go to bed with the bedroom windows wide open, only to find snow blowing in through those windows in the morning.

Well, maybe it's not quite that extreme, but it sometimes seems that way.

As for me, I've always been a summer person. I don't really enjoy intense heat and humidity, but I prefer it to bone-chilling cold and blizzards. I especially love the long daylight hours of summer. I start getting dejected on June 22, when the days begin getting shorter. And I HATE it when the stores start advertising "back-to-school" specials a week after schools have closed for the summer. Then they compound the offense by hauling out the Halloween decorations on August 1. Isn't the death of July disheartening enough? Do they have to remind me that October (the last month of the year when, with a little luck, we might have some nice days) will also soon be gone?

On the other hand, my friend Jane, who prefers winter, claims she not only likes the cold, she loves the darkness at 4:00 P.M. "It's cozy!" she says. Puhleeze! You know how I spell "cozy"? D-E-P-R-E-S-S-I-N-G! To counter the early darkness in winter, I bought a lamp that was advertised to "spread sunshine all over the room." In reality, it spreads a couple of weak beams over about one square foot of my desk.

Jane always tries to cheer me up in mid December by proclaiming that the days will be getting longer and spring will soon arrive. That just dejects me more. Spring means another birthday for me, and I don't need a reminder that another one is swooping down on me.

My friend Irma hates summer because she dislikes being confined indoors with air conditioning. What about being cooped up indoors with artificial heat all winter? At least the summer heat doesn't restrict your activities. You can go to the movies, shopping, for a walk, whatever. Not so in winter when snow and ice make driving impossible (if you can ever shovel out your car, that is) and walking perilous. The mere thought of a broken hip is enough to discourage any forays beyond the front door until the first thaw.

If you are foolhardy enough to venture outside, you must deal with the whole wardrobe issue. In summer, you can just grab your car keys and go, whereas in winter you have to allot at least twenty minutes to layering—T-shirt, turtleneck, sweatshirt, parka, knit hat (with ear flaps), woolen scarf, mittens, . . . and that's just the top half of your body. Below the waist come the tights, long johns, woolen socks, ski pants, and boots. By the time you've put all these on, you're already late for wherever you were going. Furthermore, you look like Sasquatch and you can't move.

If you ever do make it out, returning home is equally traumatic. You must remove the boots before you even step over the threshold, or the stuff you had put on your walk to melt the ice will eat a hole through your carpet and/or floor. And what to do with the rest of your outer clothing? Forget hanging them in the mudroom, if you have one. You haven't shoveled out a path to the back door, remember?

But not to worry, your front hall or living room will become a mudroom as you divest yourself of all those ice-caked layers, which start dripping over everything as soon as they hit the heated interior of your house (unless the furnace has conked out again, that is).

My winter-loving friends claim that tracking beach sand into the house in summer is just as bad. Hah! Not even close. First, you can shake the sand out of your sandals at the door since your toes will not get frostbitten while you do. And should any get inside, two minutes with a broom or vacuum cleaner takes care of it. No need to send a distress call to Carpet Catastrophes 'R Us.

Furthermore, in summer you have no expensive dry-cleaning bills. You just toss all those cotton-blend shirts, skirts, shorts, and slacks into the machine and press the wash 'n' wear cycle button. Imagine all the closet space you'd have if you didn't have to store bulky winter coats, jackets, sweaters, and boots.

As for your hair, though it may frizz up in the heat and humidity, that's more attractive than the flat hat-hair you must endure all winter because of those aforementioned knit caps.

The winter worshippers rhapsodize that all these inconveniences are a small price to pay for the beauty of the sun sparkling on a carpet of new-fallen snow. In the backyard, maybe. The front, however, unless you live in Sherwood Forest, is another story. Within an hour after a storm, the exhausts of passing cars transform the glistening mounds into dirty, dismal, disgusting glop.

It's fortunate that though we can talk about the weather endlessly, we can't do anything about it. Politicians have enough to squabble over without adding climate control to the mix. Candidates used to promise such things as "a chicken in every pot." I couldn't be that easily bought. But guarantee me a little grass shack on a sunny Hawaiian beach, and my vote is yours.

Beyond My Wildest Dreams

I just read about a truck driver who hit the lottery for $250 million dollars.

Whoopee! No more fighting traffic. No more trying to stay awake on those overnight hauls. No more driving through rain, sleet, and snow to meet delivery deadlines.

Well, not exactly. This particular truck driver loves his job and does not plan to give it up.

Is he crazy? Would you do the same? Not me.

If I had won a humongous lottery when I was working, the first thing I would have done (after writing my letter of resignation) is renew my passport. Next, I would have made reservations to travel (luxury class this time) to all my favorite locales I visited before on the cheap—first in the U.S., from the rocky coast of Maine to the hills of San Francisco and all the spectacular places in between. Then Rome, Venice, Capri, London, Dublin, Zermatt, Paris, all those sweet little towns along the Rhine in Germany, Copenhagen, Stockholm, the fiords of Norway, Mexico, Rio, Canada, the beautiful islands of Hawaii. Ditto the Caribbean. After that, I would have set my sights on countries I have never seen, from Australia to Zimbabwe.

Today, though, I would probably scale back those plans. Now that I'm older, all that traveling might be a bit taxing, despite the first-class flights, limos, and deluxe five-star accommodations I'd demand. I guess I'd have to be realistic and mind my ABCs— arthritis, bursitis, colitis . . .

So I'd probably stick closer to home. A new abode, of course. One with enough closets—finally! In fact, I might consider building two adjoining homes with a connecting indoor walkway. I'd fit two of the rooms in the second home with mirrored walls and racks. One would hold all my winter clothes and another my summer togs (all with designer labels, of course). No more seasonal switching! A third room would house wall-to-wall ledges for my shoes, and I'd divide the other rooms into storage nooks and crannies for all those items now crammed under my beds and on the floors of my crowded closets—luggage, extra blankets, pillows, holiday decorations, vacuum cleaners, umbrellas, beach chairs, gift-wrapping materials, unwanted gifts to be regifted . . .

In my living quarters, I'd equip the kitchen with state-of-the-art appliances, and it would be large enough to accommodate not merely an island, but maybe a small continent. Oh, what the heck, why not a large continent? In addition to several large bedrooms, each with its own luxury bath and dressing room, I'd also demand a spacious living room (think the Great Hall at Versailles); a dining room with a table for thirty, instead of the four guests I'm presently limited to; and a room that would serve as *only* my office—and not also have to double (or rather triple) as a den and guest quarters. Of course, it would have ample space to accommodate all my computer equipment, file cabinets, storage cabinets, book cases, and a pool-table-sized desk . . . and, hey, maybe a pool table, too. I don't play, but what the heck.

Needless to say (but I'll say it anyway), all of the rooms would be equipped with surround-sound music systems and gigantic wall-mounted plasma TVs that would be tastefully camouflaged and hidden from view, coming forth only when bidden.

Obviously, I'd hire a cordon-bleu chef, a cleaning staff, and a crew of landscapers to transform my surrounding acres into fantasyland.

It occurs to me that since I wouldn't be doing my own cooking and home and garden maintenance, I would need to exercise. So

I'd better add a fully equipped gym to my blueprints, complete with a hunky personal trainer. Oh, and an Olympic-sized indoor pool with retractable roof for warm, sunny days. So what if I can't swim; I'll hire someone to swim for me.

Also high on my list of priorities is a capacious garage so I wouldn't have to clean snow off my car all winter long. Come to think of it, I wouldn't need to live where it snows in winter any more! I could build duplicate living quarters on the shores of a tropical beach to which I could retreat as soon as the temperature dipped below seventy degrees.

But back to that garage. Naturally, I wouldn't leave it empty. I'd buy a new luxury car or two—every year for the next fifty. I'm not going to live that long, you say. Hey, whose fantasy is this? Furthermore, I'd look young and beautiful forever because I could afford plastic surgery to erase every wrinkle as it appeared.

Okay, okay. I admit it. This all sounds extraordinarily selfish. A more commendable plan would be to distribute my newfound wealth to worthy causes, relatives, and friends. Actually, I already have a list (that's true!); but it's not necessarily complete. If you're really good to me, I might add your name.

But you have to be nice *before* I hit the jackpot. Fawning over me afterwards doesn't count.

'Til Death Do Us Part . . . or Not

My friend Sarah pounded on my door last night, sobbing uncontrollably.

"Sarah?" I asked. "What's wrong?"

She blubbered incoherently as I led her into the living room where she crumpled onto the couch. I had never seen Sarah—or anyone—so upset. Obviously, something tragic had happened. I hugged her, trying to calm her.

"What is it? Tell me!"

She only cried louder.

"Is something wrong with one of the kids?" I asked.

She shook her head wildly, spraying tears.

"Not one of the grandkids?" I tried again.

"No," she finally managed to blurt. "It's Dan."

"Oh, my God!" I said. "What happened?" I could imagine only the worst. An accident? A fatal mugging? "Is he dead?" I gulped

"Not yet," she wailed, "but soon."

I hugged her again. "Oh, sweetie, what is it? Cancer? His heart?"

"No," she said, suddenly coherent and seething. "A bullet to the brain. I'm going to kill him!"

Dan and Sarah were the ideal couple, the ones the rest of us openly envied. The romance had never gone out of their marriage. Dan marked every anniversary with a beautiful gift and an original poem. He sent Sarah flowers not only on her birthday, but also on the birthdays of their three children, and even on February 2—to celebrate the beginning of spring if the groundhog didn't see his shadow, or to cheer Sarah up about the prospect of six more weeks of winter if he did.

Just last week, we had all been invited to their fortieth wedding anniversary party. At dinner, Dan apologized to Sarah that his present for her wouldn't be ready until next week. However, he assured her it was worth waiting for.

Our imaginations went wild: The Jaguar she had been coveting? The sable coat he had been promising for years to buy her "some day"? A flawless Tiffany diamond? Or maybe a round-the-world cruise in the honeymoon suite of the *Queen Mary 2?*

Rumors were rampant, fueled mainly by Sarah herself who called me daily with new speculations, including all the above and more. She was even more excited than a five-year-old waiting for Santa's visit.

And now she was threatening homicide? Quite a leap. Could Dan's "surprise" have been a cruel announcement that he was leaving her for another woman—or maybe another man? Impossible. I'd find it easier to believe that Columbus's discovery that the world is round had been a hoax and that we were all in danger of falling off the edge of the planet.

I poured Sarah some brandy and forced her to take several sips.

"Okay," I said when she had regained some composure. "What in heaven's name is going on?"

"My wonderful surprise gift," she fumed. "It didn't come in a big box. It didn't come in a little box. It came in an envelope!"

So that was it. Dan had given her a gift certificate—a very generous one, I was certain, so she could buy the present of her dreams. Maybe a copout that requires little thought, but still . . .

"I know how you feel, honey," I said, "but a gift certificate isn't a motive for murder."

"No," Sarah corrected. "Not a gift certificate. A deed!"

Had he bought a new house for them? It must be far away for

Sarah to be this distraught. Now I was getting upset, too. I love Sarah and Dan. I would miss them.

Maybe it was just a vacation getaway, a condo in the Outer Banks, a *pied-à-terre* in Paris, a penthouse in Manhattan for theater weekends. Was she upset because he had made such an important commitment without consulting her first to determine her preference?

"A deed for a second home?" I ventured hopefully.

"Oh, it's a deed for a home, all right," fumed Sarah, chug-a-lugging the rest of her brandy. "But not a second home! Our final home!"

"Huh?"

"It's a deed to a cemetery plot!" she cried. And that's not all. He also prepaid our funerals! The nerve of him."

"Well, actually, that's very thoughtful," I rationalized. "I think it's a great idea."

It was Sarah's turn to say, "Huh?" She didn't buy it. She said they had plenty of time to plan for their eventual demise. Right now, she said, she would have definitely preferred the Jaguar, the sable, the diamond, a vacation home . . .

"How can you say it's a great idea?" she demanded.

"I mean it," I said. "None of us likes to think about the inevitable, Sarah; and now you don't have to. You can relax and enjoy the rest of your life. Actually, it's a very thoughtful gift. I think it's sweet."

"Sweet?" she exploded. "I don't believe you. Maybe in ten or twenty years. What's his damn hurry?"

"And the worst part is," she continued. "He has the nerve to be disappointed in *me*. He thought I'd love it. He said nothing could be more romantic than a gift that ensures we'll be lying side by side for eternity."

I don't know about eternity, but I have a distinct feeling that Sarah and Dan won't be sharing a resting place again on this side of the Pearly Gates until he puts that plot and those prepaid funerals up for sale on eBay and uses the proceeds for a spectacular appeasement gift.

No, I'm not talking nursing home insurance.

The Buzz about Bees

In the fashion world, brown is the new black; on the health and beauty front, sixty is the new forty; and on the scholastic scene, a spelling bee is the new Big Game, and a champion speller now outshines the star quarterback or homecoming queen.

Who would have ever believed that knowing how to spell "chiaroscurist," "xanthosis," or "pickelhaube" could earn someone not only an "A" in English, but also national acclaim, and, even more important, the admiration and envy of his or her peers? It's the classic revenge of the nerds:

"Yes, Bix, I know you were elected the Handsomest Homeroom Hunk and that you kicked the winning field goal that won the championship for Cornhusk High for the first time in twenty years, but I'm going to the prom with Wilbur. He can spell "vivisepulture."

For almost two hundred years, spelling bees, which originated in the early 1800s, were the domain of brainy, and therefore unpopular, kids. Recently, however, the contests have become so cool that ESPN annually televises the Super Bowl of bees—the Scripps finals.

Even Broadway and Hollywood have latched onto the craze, turning out hit shows and movies featuring spelling bees, a concept that sounds like box office poison, but instead is breaking records. Go figure.

It is ironic that spelling bees have become so popular in an age where misspellings are not only tolerated, but they proliferate—i.e.,

"Boyz'n da Hood," "phat farm," "C U later," "R U there?," "gangsta," "ho" (I'm not talking gardening tools here), "What's ur sign?," and thousands of other abominable abbreviations that confront us daily in our newspapers and magazines and on television screens, highway billboards, and especially our computer monitors. We foolishly rely on spell-check programs that will allow us to type something like, "I went two the store too buy to pounds of hamburger." All the words are spelled correctly, so we don't bother to question whether the computer has checked for context. In addition, the informality of e-mail seems to have given us license to corrupt the language mercilessly, fostering a completely new vocabulary of *phractured* phrases and phonetic *phantasies.*

At the opposite side of the spectrum, the regulations for spelling bees are more stringent than Robert's Rules of Order. Could this be God's way of evening things up?

Admit it. Isn't it refreshing to know that some kids busily study word lists for hours each night instead of sitting at their computers divulging their real names, addresses, and anatomical measurements to an online sexual predator or trying to outgun the Super Mario Brothers?

And how about seeing these kids conservatively dressed and neatly coiffed as they respectfully ask an adult, "Could you use that word in a sentence, please?"

It's like 1940 all over again. None of the girls (including the prematurely well-developed ones) are wearing skintight, spaghetti-strapped, plunging-neckline camisoles; and not even one boy sports low-slung, baggy jeans or a T-shirt with an X-rated slogan. Who knew spelling bees could accomplish such miracles?

Adults are also jumping up on the spelling stage. My town is one of thousands throughout the country that hold annual bees where teams from various organizations compete with each other. Last year I was recruited to join three other women from my senior center to form a team. We were pitted against town teachers, retailers, business executives, and young homemakers.

It wasn't pretty. We went down in the second round. We misspelled "misspell." For days, we had studied lists of difficult words (I was even prepared to spell "supercalifragilisticexpialidocious") only to be tripped up by such a simple word. Oh, the ignominy! (Sure, that one I can spell. Unfortunately, it wasn't one of the words thrown at us.) Red-faced, we resorted to the handy excuse that we all had had a senior moment, and we fled the stage and ducked out of the auditorium before the house lights came up.

After that experience, I'm thinking of applying for a position as a writer of TV captions for the hearing impaired. Even with my limited abilities, I could do a better job than what's being done currently. Case in point—within less than five minutes this morning, I noted the following gaffes:

He/She Actually Said	**The Caption Read**
She found *solace* in	She found *sliss* in
I'm ready to *meet* my son	I'm ready to *heat* my son
He *cited* an *unnamed* source	He *sited* an *inane* source

Obviously, there's plenty of room for improvement. I'm ready for the challenge. By comparison with the present transcribers, I'm sure my performance would be supercalifragilisticexpialidocious.

Give Me Strength

When I signed up for a twice-weekly women's strength-training class at my senior center, I figured "piece of cake." After all, I'm in relatively good shape, no major aches, pains, or respiratory problems. I could certainly keep up with all those other middle-aged women. (Yes, I said "middle-aged." Isn't the average life span 140+?)

I walked into my first class and selected equipment from the communal box—some rubber tubing and a heavy elastic band, whose purposes I couldn't guess, and weights. Problem. There were none heavier than three pounds in the box. What kind of challenge would they provide? I'd have to buy my own five and ten pounders. But since I had no choice for this class, I had to settle for three-pound weights.

Our instructor told us to put down all our equipment, and then she hit "Play" on her mini boom box. As some bouncy music rang out, she started our warm-up with some very elementary left-right side steps. Please! I felt I was back in kindergarten dance class. (No cracks; I do remember kindergarten.)

Then she added crisscross arm swings. Suddenly, I wasn't so smug. Sure, I could do the side steps; and sure, I could do the arm swings. But together? Not easy for someone as uncoordinated as I am. No big deal, I figured. I wasn't here for lessons in grace. Bring on the exercise!

They're right when they warn, "Be careful what you ask for, you might get it," as I discovered during the next few weeks. Agony! We did bicep curls, standing wall pushups, inner and outer thigh leg lifts, knee extensions, quadricep stretches, overhead tricep bends, squats, lunges, and more. We learned what those innocent-looking rubber bands and tubing were. Instruments of torture, that's what. We wrapped the bands around our ankles when doing leg lifts to provide more resistance to our movements (God forbid it should be too easy), and the tubing added torment to a variety of other exercises. Every muscle screamed. Every joint creaked. But none of us complained. We couldn't. We were too busy concentrating on breathing. Not breathing correctly. Just gasping.

As for those three-pound weights, I quickly discarded them. I could barely lift the two pounders.

I had to make a real effort to get out of bed and drag myself to class at dawn every Wednesday and Friday, but I did. Hey, it was paid for. I was going to get there even if it killed me. And I had every reason to believe it might.

It hasn't yet, and I've been sticking it out for several months now. Has it gotten easier? I'd say no, because I'm still in agony during every class. However, I now achieve the same level of excruciating discomfort using three-pound weights instead of the lighter ones, so I guess that's progress. And I'm happy to report that I've gained weight. Why is that good? Because it obviously means I'm developing muscles. Muscles weigh more than fat, after all; and I can't possibly have added that much more fat . . . can I? Please, *please* tell me that the extra girth around my abdomen and waist is all muscle! Sure it is.

Unfortunately, despite all the triceps raises and bends, the flesh on the back of my arms still flaps in the breeze; but I have developed impressive biceps. Not only can I see and feel them when I flex, but I can now carry twenty groceries bags—ten strung on each arm—up the twenty-one steps to my condo. A mixed blessing. By doing this all in one trip, I'm strengthening my biceps still further, but I'm eliminating some stair-climbing exercise.

As for the squats, lunges, and leg extensions, my knees now

feel ninety years old. A big improvement. They used to feel 120.

An interesting feature of my strength-training class is that we have two instructors who alternate days. I think they're playing good cop/bad cop. On Wednesdays, Nancy the "Good" sneakily plays tapes of Strauss waltzes and 1940 show tunes, falsely leading us to believe the workouts will be effortless. Hah! And on Fridays, Barbara the "Bad" (and I mean that in the best possible way) puts us through our paces to a background of no-nonsense heavy metal. But they both achieve the same end result—our utter exhaustion and relief when the class is over—as well as awe and admiration for them because they both teach another group immediately following ours. That means they go through the same grueling routine twice! How do they do that?

I know what motivates me—I want to get in good enough shape to take the tap-dancing class offered by the senior center. I figure I'll be ready when my knees feel seventy-five years old.

Meanwhile, I should look into the needlework class. On second thought, maybe not. My eyes feel 150.

What's in a Name?

"What's in a name?" Shakespeare asked. "That which we call a rose by any other name would smell as sweet," said he.

True. At least in my case, because I'm sure I would have showered regularly and splashed on a little cologne occasionally, even if I wasn't called Rose.

But if my parents had named me for a more hostile flower— say, the carnivorous Venus flytrap or the poisonous plumeria— would I still have been agonizingly passive and shy throughout my childhood, adolescence, and even young adulthood; or would I have become more aggressive and assertive, qualities which, as Rose, I didn't develop until my forties?

It's not such a farfetched possibility. If I had been born today to celebrity parents, I could indeed have been named Venus Flytrap or Plumeria—which would have been much kinder than some of the wacky names celebs saddle their kids with.

I think it started more than three decades ago when singer/ musician Frank Zappa named his son Dweezil and his daughter Moon Unit. Shouldn't he have been reported to the Society against Cruelty to Children? Dweezil, in itself, is bizarre enough; but its similarity to Dweeb makes it even more offensive. Or maybe not. The Dweezil in question here, who is following in his father's musical footsteps, claims that what he himself describes as his "goofy" name is an advantage, since people always remember him because of it. I haven't heard what Moon Unit thinks of her completely senseless moniker, but since she never changed it when she became the legal age to do so, I assume she doesn't hate it. Why not, only heaven knows.

There were many periods during which celebrities' offspring were blessed with normal names—Deborah, Alan, Wendy, Steven. In fact, so ordinary and familiar were the forenames of the era that when Judy Garland named one of her daughters Liza, the "Z" instead of an "S" was considered pretty avant-garde.

Later came Sonny and Cher's daughter, Chastity. Wasn't that asking for trouble? The only way she could live that down was not to live up to it. Though maybe it worked in reverse, because I've never read about Chastity Bono's sexual indiscretions. At least not with men. And now she (or rather he) *is* a man named Chaz. Would that have happened if she had been named Jane or Mary at birth?

These aberrations pale, however, when compared with the latest rash of outlandish names today's stars inflict on their kids, including Shiloh Nouvel Jolie-Pitt. Why would Angelina and Brad name their baby after a Civil War battle and then complicate it with the hyphenated addition? I'll give you odds she'll probably be in college before she learns to spell the whole thing. And when she marries, will she drop the Jolie-Pitt or keep it and append her husband's surname with yet another hyphen?

But Shiloh (even with the hyphen) isn't as bad as Audio Science, the child of actress Shannyn (why not Shannon?) Sossamon. Maybe she'll call her next kid Video Technology.

Then there's Banjo, the son/daughter (who knows which?) of actress Rachel Griffiths. Will she name a future child Bassoon or maybe Xylophone?

Singer Toni Braxton named her children Denim and Diezel. Could be worse, I suppose. She could have chosen Burlap and Regular Unleaded.

Gwyneth Paltrow's Apple may some day have a sibling named iMac or Pomegranate (depending on whether Mom chooses to go the high-tech or fruit route).

The names Dixie Dot and Bibi Belle, daughters of British TV personality Anna Ryder Richardson, might not raise a rebel flag in Georgia or the Carolinas, but I'm sure they raise eyebrows across the pond in Trafalgar Square and Notting Hill.

Do you suppose Live Aid founder Bob Geldof and Paula Yates (another U.K. television personality) named their children Fifi Trixibell, Peaches Honeyblossom, and Pixie for the poodles or Shih Tzus they would have preferred?

Maybe God'Iss Love, daughter of rapper Lil' Mo, was named after her mother—they do share an apostrophe. Is she called God for short? Does the name mean Goddess Love (a huge potential problem when the kid hits puberty)? Or is it simply a misspelling of God is Love?

Other kids who are destined never to win the Scripps Spelling Bee are Pilot Inspektor, son of actor Jason Lee, and Reign Beau, daughter of actor Ving Rhames.

A boy who hopefully will not let his name (or his mother's occupation) determine his future profession is Pirate, son of Korn frontman Jonathan Davis and his porn-star wife, Devon.

And wasn't director Robert Rodriguez tempting fate when he named his sons Rebel and Rogue?

Jermaine Jackson dubbed his son Jermajesty, possibly an attempt to carry on the royal dynasty initiated by brother Michael, who named not one, but *both* of his sons Prince Michael. Now there's an identity crisis just waiting to happen. It's hard enough for siblings to share toys; expecting them to share the same name is disastrous, as if they won't have enough trouble trying to live down their father's reputation.

Clearly, Chef Jamie Oliver must have been guzzling the cooking sherry when he named his children Poppy Honey and Daisy Boo.

You probably think I made all these names up. Not true! I found them all documented in an Internet search . . . speaking of which, I'm surprised that no one has yet named a child Google or Yahoo.

Come on, people! Think. These kids are going to have to go

through school, play with other children, and grow up and get jobs. How are their names going to sound in the classroom, in the playground, in the boardroom? How will they look on a degree, on a résumé, on an office door? Won't these children's career choices be limited? I foresee serious problems, unless they aspire to join Barnum & Bailey or become rock stars or strippers. Let's face it. Would you want your first grader to be introduced to spelling by Miss Reign Beau or Mr. Pilot Inspektor? Would you trust your root canal or gall bladder surgery to Dr. Daisy Boo? Would you buy stock in a company headed by CEO Peaches Honeyblossom?

These crazy names will haunt their owners all their lives—and beyond. Fifi Trixibell is going to look pretty silly on a tombstone.

I'm sure glad mine will say Rose instead of Venus Flytrap.

Give Me a Break

Uncle! I give up!

I swear I'm going to stop reading newspapers and magazines, and no more TV news for me either. I simply can't take one more tale about the sufferings of my fellow man and woman.

Until now, I had been barely managing to cope with reports of suicide bombings, mass murder, and mayhem; but this morning I read something that pushed me over the edge. It was an article about a corporate executive whose compensation has been slashed by two-thirds, and he is now going to have to support himself and his family on a mere five million dollars annually.

It's inhumane. He may actually be forced to eat prime rib occasionally instead of filet mignon. Uggh! Furthermore, he may have to sell his twenty-five-room villa on Lake Como, the beachfront estate on Palm Beach, and maybe even his private island off the coast of Fiji. (I don't know that he actually owns all this real estate, but I wouldn't be surprised.)

Where will he go now to escape from the rigors of the corporate jungle—the private jet business flights, the chauffeured limousines, the thousand-dollar expense-account dinners, the bowing and scraping of his acolytes, and the countless other onerous burdens of his demanding position. It makes me want to cry. Or vomit.

His is just one tale. Fortunately, many corporate head honchos manage their businesses competently and benevolently, but the pages of *Fortune* and the *Wall Street Journal* abound with accounts of other big-biz bigwigs who are paid obscene bucks, even during periods when they cause their companies and stockholders to lose mega-millions and thousands of their employees to lose their jobs. Yet Mr. CEO apparently doesn't see anything wrong with this picture. If the "little people" have to be sacrificed, so be it—as long as all his perks and ill-gotten gains are protected. (I say "Mr." and "his" not because women are necessarily more principled, but because very few females achieve CEO-dom.)

What's really surprising is that several of these misguided captains of industry had humble beginnings—sort of the modern-day equivalent of Abe Lincoln and the log cabin. The only difference is that Abe remained humble and compassionate, even after becoming president of the United States. Not so of some of today's rags-to-riches tycoons. With every step up the corporate ladder, their grasp on reality loosens a bit more until they actually believe they are as important as their sycophants tell them they are. They develop God complexes and feel no one should have the audacity to question their authority or their motives. The board of directors demands accountability and wants to bring in outside auditors? How dare they! The stockholders are getting restless? Off with their heads!

What's with these guys? How do they get off feeling so entitled? Would I react the same in their position? I certainly hope not, but who knows? I have to admit that when I repair a tear in my two-dollar shower-curtain liner with Scotch tape, I can't possibly be objective about a corporate mogul who buys a $6,000 shower curtain (for the maid's quarters).

I'm willing to be fair. I'll be happy to accept a position as monarch of a multinational conglomerate at an annual salary that could feed a third-world country for a decade, adopt a suitably lavish lifestyle, and then see how I react if people criticize me when my mismanagement and extravagant spending drown the company in a flood of red ink. Just one year. That's all I ask.

Then I promise to resign and forfeit any future compensation.

But I do hope they'll let me keep the villa on Lake Como . . . and, of course, a generous pension. After all, by then I will have become accustomed to an opulent standard of living, and it would be heartless to expect me to give it up. How could I survive without caviar and champagne?

For now, though, I'll just settle for some sugar to sprinkle on my sour grapes.

My Amazing Journey

I've just returned from the most amazing journey!

Suddenly, I sound like all those people on so-called reality dating shows. Have you ever noticed that they all use the same script? Everything is "amazing," as in,

"This was the most amazing date of my life!"

"She/he is such an amazing girl/guy!!"

"Her/his family is so amazing!!!"

All summed up by, "This has been an amazing journey!!!!"

Yes, it's always a "journey," never simply an experience. And, yes, they do always speak with multiple explanation points.

But I digress. (I'm allowed to at my age.) Back to my own amazing journey! Unfortunately, I didn't share it with a bunch of handsome hunks or even average Joes. I traveled alone; but my journey was amazing, nevertheless. What made it so amazing? (If I don't go back to a strict PBS diet soon, I will need an emergency vocabulary transplant.) Sorry, I'm digressing again, aren't I?

Okay, I'm ready to tell you about my unusual voyage (see, I do know other words!). I zoomed from Antarctica to the tropics in just forty-eight hours. What's more, I didn't have to go through airport security, I didn't have to bother with luggage, and I didn't suffer jet lag. How come? Because I experienced these diverse environments in the comfort (or, rather, *dis*comfort) of my own New England condo.

Last Sunday night, when the temperatures dipped (how come

temperatures always dip and never simply fall?) below zero, my heat gave one last gasp and conked out. As the wind whistled outside, the baseboards in every room turned to ice. (Well, not literally, but you know what I mean.)

It was 11:00 P.M. I could have sent for the on-call weekend-emergency maintenance guy, but I hated to bother him at that hour. I'm one of those independent people who'd rather die than inconvenience anyone. Of course, I didn't realize that dying was a distinct possibility until I heard the next morning that a man in Philadelphia had succumbed to hypothermia in his sleep because he had no heat in his house. In fact, so blissfully unaware of the danger was I that I even took a sleeping pill to get me through the night, but not before I had piled every blanket and afghan I owned on my bed, plus a storm coat that guaranteed protection to temperatures of twenty degrees below zero. I had bought it last year so I'd be able to walk my daily two miles throughout the winter. (Right. I abandoned that resolution at the first sign of frost, subzero coat notwithstanding.)

Regrettably, I don't own any warm sleepwear. I prefer a cool (but not Arctic) bedroom and lots of blankets, but I can't stand flannel PJs. Apparently I'm hot in bed. (Wishful thinking.) At any rate, I wear sleeveless cotton nightgowns all year round, and this frigid night was no exception. Nevertheless, my well-blanketed cocoon protected me.

Unlike that unfortunate man in Philadelphia, I did wake up in the morning and ran from my bed to a steaming shower (thank God I still had hot water). I then donned sweat pants, a turtleneck, a heavy sweater, and my storm coat, and I called my maintenance guy who scolded me for not calling him sooner. He diagnosed my problem as a broken valve and declared I'd have to call a plumber to replace it. Meanwhile, he could patch up the valve so I would have heat, but I wouldn't be able to regulate it, so it would get very hot.

"Just open a window," he advised

Naturally, every plumber within a one-hundred-mile radius was busy fixing pipes that had burst through the night, so I was going to have to wait until the following afternoon for service. No problem, thought I. I'd be fine.

But then the heat came on full blast. I was not fine. The temperature soared. As I gasped for breath, my phone rang. It was a friend who thought I was still in the deep freeze calling to quip, "Rose, I see Wal-Mart is having a special on blankets. Shall I go get you a couple?"

"No, thanks," I said, "but I'd appreciate a bikini, if they have any."

Right, as if I could wear a bikini. More self-deception.

I did strip down to my underwear, but I did not follow my maintenance man's advice to open a window. I opened *all* my windows—wide. I turned on my ceiling fans. My house still felt like the tropics. So I decided to go with it.

I put a calypso CD in my stereo, turned my sound machine onto "surf," poured myself a gin and tonic (but had to do without a paper umbrella), sank into my recliner, closed my eyes, and imagined that the blades of the overhead fan were palm fronds stirring in an ocean breeze.

It worked fairly well for a few minutes (actually, until I finished the gin and tonic), and then reality and near heat prostration set in. I had a miserably uncomfortable night.

My plumber is due in five hours. I'm waiting for him on my icy front steps, with the wind howling around me. It feels amazing!

Bon Appétit!

Are you as confused as I am by all the admonitions about healthy eating? Read one book or news article on the subject and I guarantee it will directly contradict something you read the day before. Take the whole issue of water, for example. For decades, I've been conscientiously struggling to down eight glasses a day, and now "they" tell us we don't need to do that.

Could it be possible that what I thought was flab is simply bloat and that if I cease guzzling water, I may once again be svelte? What good news, except for the bottled water industry. (Is it too late to dump my Evian stock?)

As for the food advice, though some of the suggestions may be sound nutritionally, they are often far from practical. For example, I just read a book about foods that fight disease; and I swear, if you try to follow its guidelines, you'll be penniless in no time—for two reasons: First, you'll spend a fortune on the recommended foods; and, second, you'll have to quit your job and devote all your time to grocery shopping and eating.

Not only will you be broke, you'll also be fat and alone: Fat because of the calorie content of the amount of recommended foods and alone because your family will run away from home and all your friends will avoid you. Let's face it. Who wants to watch you stuffing your face all day, which is what you'd have to do in order to consume the required quantities of foods the book in question deems are essential, including:

Blueberries: One to two cups a day. This may be doable during the summer (especially if you have your own blueberry bushes), but to buy that many out of season, you would probably have to refinance your home because somebody (i.e., you) has to pay the shipping charges from Chile or wherever. And even if you love blueberries, how long do you think you'd continue to love them if you scarfed down two cups daily?

Pumpkin: A half-cup most days. I may be wrong, but don't pumpkins have an even shorter season than blueberries?

Spinach: One cup steamed or two cups raw most days. Come on! Even Popeye didn't eat that much.

Wild salmon: Two to four times per week. If you can't find salmon in the wild, it's going to cost you last month's pension check at the fish market.

Tomatoes: One serving per day of processed tomatoes and multiple servings per week of fresh tomatoes. Okay, so a daily salad would take care of the fresh tomatoes requirement; but that one serving per day of processed tomatoes is problematic. What are you going to put it on? Pasta? Pizza? Every day? How do you spell "e-x-p-a-n-d-i-n-g waistline"?

Yogurt: Two cups daily. Give me a break! When are we supposed to fit this in? I suppose we could mix some of it with the blueberries and spread the rest on some stewed tomatoes or steamed spinach.

Soy: At least fifteen grams of soy protein each day. I'm not sure what soy protein is, but I do know that fifteen grams must be a lot because you're supposed to divide it into two separate meals or snacks.

Oats or other grains such as brown and wild rice, barley, wheat germ, and flaxseed: Five to seven servings a day! Follow this suggestion, and you'll be neighing in no time.

Oh, let's not forget that daily apple that will keep the doctor away. Right, like keeping the doctor away is a problem these days. When was the last time one came knocking on your door?

In addition, the following are recommended: A half-cup to one cup of broccoli and an orange every day, at least four servings of beans per week, an ounce of walnuts five times a week, and three to four servings of turkey breast per week.

Keep in mind that all of the above are touted in just one book. Other sources specify even more essential nutrients. The last time I checked, a week still had only seven days. So how are you supposed to fit everything into a daily meal plan? And what happens when you dine out? Won't you get some strange looks when you order two cups of blueberries, a cup of yogurt, and half a cup of pumpkin for dinner?

Most important, where do ice cream and Scotch fit into this scheme? How can a diet be well balanced without these two essentials?

Then there's the whole issue of nutritional supplements. How are we going to manage to swallow (and pay for) all the vitamins and minerals supposedly required daily to keep us healthy, gorgeous, and pain free? It's a challenge. Some must be taken with food, others at least an hour before or after eating, some in the morning, some at bedtime, and some on alternate Thursdays, except when the moon is full. Okay, so I made the last one up; but you know what I mean.

Add to this mix potions for controlling stomach upset (which is guaranteed if you consume all of the above); pills for heartburn (ditto); capsules to help block carbohydrates (a must if you're going to eat all the pizza and pasta to use as a base for your daily required processed tomatoes); laxatives for irregularity; and magic tablets to cure everything from social anxiety disorder (formerly known as plain old shyness) to attention deficit disorder (i.e., formerly called boredom and/or rambunctiousness) to a wide range of male and female sexual dysfunctions (formerly never mentioned in public, unlike today when celebrities freely admit their inadequacies on national TV and magazine ads).

I'd like to stay and discuss this further, but I must go. It's time to force myself to eat my wild salmon and soy casserole.

If It Sounds too Good to Be True

I got such a bargain a while back, a Web camera for only $4.74, after in-store and mail-in rebates. It was so unbelievable, I bought two—one for me and one for my niece Shelley who lives in Syracuse, New York, 250 miles away, so when her adorable children, Madeline, Alexandra, and Jonathan, blow me kisses over the phone, I'd actually be able to see them through the magic of Skype. Technology—it's wonderful.

Or not.

I filled out the registration form for my camera; then, to save Shelley the time, I also registered hers before sending it to her, which was not easy. One of the blanks to be filled in was the camera's serial number, which was etched in faint, miniscule characters on a translucent, light-reflecting panel smack on top of an intricate circuit board. A half-hour and two magnifying glasses later, I managed to decipher the numbers.

I then attempted to install my camera. Another problem: the accompanying leaflet that masqueraded as a manual was about as helpful as a paper parasol in a monsoon. So I winged it. I studied the camera. So cute! (I'm a sucker for miniature electronic devices.) I figured out how to connect its cable to a USB port in my computer. Drunk with success, I then inserted the software—a floppy disk and a CD-ROM that refused to run until I begged St. Jude, the patron saint of impossible causes, to intercede.

Finally, an encouraging display appeared on my monitor. I

clicked on various headings, and another window popped up with a graphic of a small TV screen. Now what? One of the buttons on the display was a question mark. It was reading my mind. I clicked on the question mark, and it linked me to online instructions—more than fifty pages of links and superlinks that had to be accessed separately. I printed them all out—twice—one for me and one for Shelley, resulting in the premature death of a $28 printer cartridge; but what the heck. Seeing Maddie, Allie, and Johnny—in addition to hearing them—would be worth every penny.

These images inspired me to take a break from my installation activity and rush to the post office to send Shelley her camera and instructions printout—Priority Mail, $8.50—but I'm not complaining.

Then back home to finish installing my own Web cam. Four hours later (I'm not exaggerating), I still hadn't succeeded. I kept getting error messages: "The video capture device is in use. Please close the application that is using video capture and retry." No other applications were running. I had no idea what this meant.

Another message popped up: "There was a problem contacting the conexs.com server."

Huh? I gamely (spelled s-t-u-p-i-d-l-y) kept at it. Two hours later (still not kidding), I decided to uninstall the program, go to bed, and start again from scratch after a good night's sleep.

Right. Like I could sleep.

At 3:00 A.M., I got up, turned on my computer, fired off a "Help!" message to the camera manufacturer's technical support e-mail address, then tackled the installation again. I was still at it at 7:00 A.M. (true; I swear). By now, I had not only not installed the camera, but I had managed to mess up my entire system. I could no longer connect to my e-mail, and I couldn't even shut off my computer properly—I had to do it by turning off the power (a big NO-NO in computerland).

Fortunately, I was able to revert the system to a selected previous time. I set it to go back twenty-four hours, before the

Web cam madness began. This restored my computer's sanity, but not mine.

Now able to connect to the Internet, I checked my e-mail and found a response from the camera manufacturer's tech support. It suggested I call an 800 number for live help to resolve my problems. I did.

After being kept on Hold Hell for forty-five minutes, listening to repeated recorded messages of praise about the company's products and services, an actual living being came on the line. I told him my problems. He said he could help. He lied. Not that he didn't try. He guided me, step by step, through various procedures. I could sense he was becoming as frustrated as I when he kept running into the same roadblocks I had encountered on my own.

Suddenly, I heard a click. He was gone. An accidental disconnect? I think not.

I called back. That's right. Hold Hell again until another techie finally answered. Different guy. Same story. Except he didn't hang up; at least not until he told me there was obviously something wrong with the camera.

"Take it back and exchange it," he suggested.

And start this exercise in futility all over again? Not on your life. Instead, I bought a new laptop with a built-in Web cam. It's great!

Now if I could only figure out how to get Skype to work.

Happy New Year!

Am I glad I didn't live in Babylonia four thousand years ago. There the New Year celebration lasted eleven days. One is bad enough.

By the eleventh day, the Babylonians must have had prodigious hangovers. They probably weren't even fully conscious for the first month of the new year. That's not for me. It would mean missing all those great postholiday sales.

I hate New Year's—the whole shebang, beginning with New Year's Eve. The forced gaiety. The pressure to be HAPPY! It's all so depressing.

When I was young, the worst part was that if I didn't have a date for New Year's Eve, it cast a pall on the next twelve months. One year, to avoid the social ignominy of being dateless on the Big Night, a girl friend and I fled to Manhattan to mingle with the throngs in Times Square so no one could tell that we were unescorted. No one, that is, except a couple of sleazy characters who latched onto us and tried to entice us back to their pad to "start the new year off with a bang."

Did we really look that desperate? When we adamantly refused, a drunk who had been eavesdropping berated us for "spoiling the boys' new year." Give me a break! That was even more disheartening than being home with the old folks watching Guy Lombardo on TV.

Now that *I'm* an "old folk," I miss Guy Lombardo; and I don't hate New Year's Eve any more because I no longer feel pressured to party. Instead, I can go to bed early and sleep through the countdown. It's wonderful!

But when I wake up, it's New Year's Day, which is not so wonderful, because I feel compelled to make those cursed resolutions that I know are doomed to failure. If I didn't lose those stubborn ten pounds last year, why will turning a page on the calendar help me shed them this year? (Could you hand me that last brownie, please? And don't be stingy with the ice cream.)

And why would I think that taking a new pledge to hike three miles a day is going to work when it never did before? It's too cold to go out and walk anyway. It's January in New England, for heaven's sake! I'll start in April when it warms up a bit. Or maybe not. What would be the point? I would have already blown three months.

Don't look at me like that. I know I really must cut down on sweets and ramp up my exercise. And I will. But making a resolution on January 1 and then giving up completely the first time I weaken isn't going to do it. Eating a hunk of cheesecake on January 3 and foregoing the three-mile walk on January 5 should not give me an excuse to stuff myself and flop on the couch every day for the rest of the year.

On the bright side, I have stuck to at least one of last year's resolutions: I've stopped wasting time playing computer Free Cell solitaire. Instead, however, I'm now addicted to computer Spider solitaire. Whenever I sit down at the computer to work that insidious game draws me into its web and traps me there for at least an hour. I'd resolve to give it up, but I'm afraid something even more obsessive will replace it.

At least I'm not smoking. But then I never smoked. So I suppose that can't be counted as a victory.

Since resolutions do often backfire and sabotage us, why do we still make them? Because we're slaves to a tradition that started way back in 153 B.C. when the Romans placed their god Janus at the head of the calendar. Janus was two-faced (no, not like the smiling backstabber you worked with ten years ago). Janus literally had two faces—one on the back of his head reviewing the old year and its disappointments, and the other on the front looking toward the incoming year with its potential for positive change.

I really must get serious about making some positive changes myself; and even though intellectually I know that New Year's resolutions usually don't work, I can't be the only person on the planet who won't make a few. So this coming year I resolve to reread all of Shakespeare's works, and not just the Cliff Notes this time; to practice the piano, and not just "Chopsticks" and "Heart & Soul"; to learn Italian, and not just the entrées on the Olive Garden menu.

Actually, I'm tempted to forget the self-improvement vows and make some resolutions that would be fun to keep like eat more chocolate, do less housework, spend more money, watch more frivolous TV shows, cut back on exercise, and sleep 'til noon. But if I did, I'm sure those resolutions would "take"; and I'd hate myself by mid January.

However, while researching resolutions around the world, I did find one associated with my Sicilian ancestry that would be easy to keep and shouldn't do too much damage: Eat lasagna on New Year's Day to ensure good fortune for the coming year. I much prefer that to the Austrian belief that good luck will flow to those who dine on suckling pig on New Year's Day, a practice that certainly isn't very lucky for the pig.

The lasagna idea has a much greater appeal. Since an entire roasted cow isn't the centerpiece on the table, I don't have to face the fact that the hamburger in the sauce was once an animal possibly named Elsie. Actually, there's no need to sacrifice Elsie. I make a scrumptious meat-free marinara sauce.

This makes the Sicilian tradition even more tantalizing— so much so that I may even adopt the ancient Babylonian custom of celebrating New Year's. Then I could enjoy lasagna for eleven days.

On second thought, an eleven-day New Year's holiday would mean eleven New Year's Eves to get through.

There isn't enough lasagna in all of Italy to make that worthwhile.

Slim Down? Fat Chance!

Obesity has become a huge problem, so to speak, not only in the United States, but also worldwide, including the Orient, where tubbiness was practically unknown, except for Japan's Sumo wrestlers, before the invasion of McDonald's and other purveyors of American junk food.

Is this international epidemic of corpulence our fault? Partly. But not entirely. In post World War II Germany, for example, portliness was desirable because it signified wealth. The more Wiener schnitzel and strudel Herr and Frau Schmidt could afford to eat, the richer they were, so they proudly paraded their poundage before their skinnier, less affluent countrymen.

During that same postwar period, well-heeled Americans indulged in expensive toys—yachts, Lamborghinis, and private planes instead of rich tortes and diamonds and designer duds instead of goulash and gesundheitwurst. They joined exclusive country clubs and worked off their champagne and caviar calories by playing golf, squash, and other games of the idle rich. They nursed tennis elbows instead of gourmand-induced gout. In short, among wealthy Americans, thin was in. "You can never be too thin or too rich" was the mantra of the day.

Not any more. Oh, we may still believe it, but it seems we've given up trying to achieve it. Why have so many of our citizens, from toddlers to tottering seniors, become so obese they can barely waddle ten steps without wheezing and whining? It isn't just because of *what* they're eating; it's also how much. Who can say no when asked, "Do you want fries with that?" (They smell so good.) Further, who can resist an offer to supersize those fries and all the other unhealthy menu choices? Is it any surprise that something called a "Whopper" is not a diet food?

And are you naïve enough to think that washing it down with a half-gallon of liquid sugar is going to flush it out of your system before it has a chance to establish a beachhead in your abdomen?

I have also noticed that no food items come in "small" any more, with one exception. A local ice cream stand actually does offer large, medium, small, *and* baby cones. I won't attempt to describe the first three choices. Suffice it to say that the "baby" cone is large enough to satisfy a baby rhino.

As for other foods, we can usually choose from "regular" (which is huge), "medium" (humongous), and "large" (roll out the wheelbarrow, Mama; you can't carry this yourself).

Even more ridiculous, today I went to my hospital for a cholesterol blood test. I then had a half-hour to kill before the time of a follow-up appointment with my doctor. Since I had fasted from the previous evening, I was hungry and decided to splurge on coffee and a bagel with cream cheese in the hospital cafeteria while I waited.

I couldn't believe what I saw. Were those really bagels on that tray? They were large and dense enough to serve as tires for a Mack truck. And since they were so hefty, I needed four packets of cream cheese just to thinly cover the entire surface. But I would eat only half, I promised myself. Of course, I broke that promise. And I didn't even enjoy it. Each guilty mouthful tasted like cardboard. But I soldiered on and ate the whole thing while praying that my doctor wouldn't insist on weighing me prior to my examination.

If this is what they're offering in the cafeterias of hospitals, which preach healthy diets, it's no wonder that commercial eateries now serve amounts of food suitable for slopping the hogs.

Case in point: A friend and I recently shared an entrée meant for one at a nearby Italian restaurant. We each ate enough pasta and meatballs to fuel us through the next week (and neither of us has a dainty appetite); and I brought home the leftovers, which provided three additional substantial meals. Crazy!

Unfortunately, as portion sizes increase, my will power decreases. This is not good. I must exercise control—or at least exercise, period. And I would, except exercise really makes me hungry. In fact, just thinking about exercise makes me hungry.

Would you pass me a tiny piece of that raspberry cheesecake, please?

Oh, what the heck—supersize it.

Eeny, Meeny, Miny, Moe

Yesterday I went shopping for a book to help me unravel the mysteries of my recently acquired digital camera. I eventually narrowed my search to either *Digital Photography for Dummies* or *The Complete Idiot's Guide to Digital Photography.* I panicked. I couldn't decide if I'm a dummy or an idiot. So I didn't buy either book. Instead, I went to lunch to relax and recover from my identity crisis.

"Would you like something to drink?" the waiter asked.

Absolutely. After all, I was there to unwind.

"Yes, please," I said. "A glass of wine."

"Which would you prefer?" he asked, handing me a leather-bound, gilt-embossed wine menu that was thicker and more intimidating than my computer manual.

I gulped.

"Perhaps I can help narrow it down," he offered, sensing my bewilderment. "First, would you like red or white?"

Another quandary. I had planned to order fish for lunch. Did that mean I should drink white wine? But isn't red better for the heart? And if I decided on a red wine, should I have steak instead of fish? But isn't red meat bad for the heart? By now, I was sure the waiter was convinced I was an idiot. Was he right? Should I go back to the bookstore and buy the idiot's digital photography guide? That's a dumb way to make a decision, I thought; so maybe I should get the dummies book . . .

Meanwhile, the waiter was shuffling from one foot to another, sighing heavily, checking his watch, then the calendar on the wall. The pressure! I couldn't take it any more. I grabbed my purse, mumbled something about an appointment I had forgotten, and fled.

Fortunately, despite my discombobulated state, I managed to find my car in the parking lot and headed for the exit. But should I turn right and drive home via the highway, or left and take the byways? I knew the highway would be clogged with traffic at that hour. On the other hand, the route via the side roads was painfully slow and tortuous.

What to do? Delay the decision, of course. Instead of going home right then, I'd go shopping. So I reversed back into the parking lot and made a beeline for Macy's. Unfortunately, once inside the store, the path I chose led me right smack into the cosmetics aisle.

Big mistake.

I was immediately accosted by an overly groomed, overly perfumed, overly solicitous beauty consultant (that's how her name badge identified her) who quickly appraised my face and launched into a spiel about a new miracle wrinkle cream that she assessed (correctly, I admit) I direly needed. Her own skin, of course, was as smooth as the proverbial baby's behind. Was it because she used the products she was touting, or because she was about forty years younger than I? In addition to the wrinkle cream, she strongly suggested I "invest" in a large jar of make-up removal scrub (when did soap and water become obsolete?), a larger jar of rich moisturizer, and a flacon of skin toner.

"Tsk! Tsk! You've really been neglecting your pores," she scolded.

She wasn't sure if I needed the "cooling revitalizing" or the "stress relieving" toner to restore my pH equilibrium, which cleansing (probably with the make-up removal scrub) could unbalance. There was a third choice, a "thirst-quenching" version with glycolic and amino acids, which she promised would remove dulling surface cells and bring a fresh radiance to my skin.

And I thought trying to decide between a white or a red wine was a challenge! I used my "forgotten appointment" excuse and scurried away, as the beauty consultant called after me, "Wait! We haven't discussed your dark circles and puffy undereyes yet!"

By now, the traffic had subsided a bit, so I hit the highway for home, but made a short detour to the supermarket. More dilemmas. Should I buy organic or regular tomatoes? Greenhouse or vine ripened? Beefsteak, plum, cherry, or grape (I'm still talking tomatoes here)? And how about apples? McIntosh? Cortland? Delicious? Granny Smith? Washington State? New York State? Empire? Fuji? Jonathan? Macoun? Northern Spy? Winesap? I settled on one of each.

Cereal. I needed cereal. But I didn't need the aggravation I encountered in the cereal aisle—shelves laden with more than thirty selections, each fortified with a different, impressive array of vitamins and minerals. I'm not a doctor. How do I choose? I used the scientific method. I closed my eyes, spun around three times, then reached out and grabbed a box. I'm sure I'll enjoy the sugar-coated oat clusters sprinkled with gummy bears.

That reminded me. Toothpaste. I was completely out. Just that morning, I learned that toothpaste has an expiration date (who knew?), and I had to throw away three tubes I had bought on sale a while back—actually *quite* a while back, judging from the staggering new assortment that had been added since my last purchase. I could now select from more than a dozen brands, each of which offered both regular and gel versions of a cavity-fighting, *or* whitening, *or* tartar control, *or* plaque removal, *or* fluoride-fortified, *or* gum disease protection formula. I need all of the above. If I opt to fight cavities, for example, will I have to sacrifice tartar control? And if I do, won't that promote cavities? Should I buy them all and use every one of them daily? Our parents and grandparents never had to choose from such a confusing variety of products. They did the job merely by sprinkling a little baking soda on a utilitarian toothbrush that didn't oscillate, rotate, or vibrate—or, in fact, involve electricity or batteries.

Today's world requires too many options, too many stress-inducing decisions. No wonder so many people are in therapy.

Hey! Maybe a few sessions on the couch could help me become more decisive. I'll just find a psychotherapist in the yellow pages. . . . Oh, no! More than three hundred are listed!

I can't deal with this right now. My head is pounding. I've got to go to the drugstore and buy some aspirin.

But, wait. Do I want tablets or capsules . . . normal or extra strength . . . plain or buffered . . .?

HELP!

How Come?

No wonder I'm an insomniac. How can I get to sleep when I keep trying to solve life's little puzzles, such as:

How come the label on my sleeping pills warns, "May cause drowsiness"? Isn't that the point? Conversely, why is my antivertigo medication marked, "May cause dizziness"?

How come when people say, "To make a long story short . . ." they never do? And invariably, when they utter the phrase, "Needless to say . . ." they say it anyway.

How come guests never use guest hand towels, even when they're prominently displayed by the bathroom sink? Have you ever noticed that after a dinner party or an afternoon of Scrabble, though several people have visited the lavatory from time to time, not one of the guest towels has been disturbed? They're still in place, pristinely folded and unrumpled. I'm giving my friends the benefit of the doubt and assuming that they do wash their hands; but apparently, they dry them on the face or bath towels on the racks, on the seat of their pants, or possibly a piece of toilet tissue. Do they think I put the guest towels out for some more important visitors I'm expecting later?

And why do we decorate our bathrooms with seashells? Is the water flowing from our faucets somehow connected to the ocean? I myself live only twenty miles from the Atlantic, so maybe the shells in my bathroom aren't so incongruous; however, I'm willing to bet that if you go into almost any bathroom in a home in, say, Kansas City, you'll also find a conch shell or two, which you can hold to your ear and listen for the sound of the surf, even though the only waves for hundreds of miles are of amber-colored grain.

Another conundrum that keeps me awake is what happens to the mattresses people return if they're not satisfied with them after a thirty-day free trial? Some of them cost several thousand dollars. Am I to believe they are destroyed and not simply recycled? If you ask me, Mama, Papa, and Baby Bear were pretty astute when they observed, "Someone's been sleeping in my bed." Did someone snooze (or worse!) in mine before me? Hand me that Lysol spray, please.

If absence makes the heart grow fonder, how can out of sight be out of mind?

And if God will provide, how come he helps only those who help themselves?

More important, why does my computer crash only when I'm behind deadline on a vital project and not when I'm playing solitaire—especially since I spend much more time playing games than working?

And can wine connoisseurs really detect undertones of leather, tea, oak, and dozens of other essences and aromas? When they describe a certain vintage as having "a good nose" or "legs," are they putting me on? And when they toss out adjectives like "assertive," "attractive," "graceful," and "elegant," are they really describing the wine or the waitress pouring it?

If haste makes waste, how come he who hesitates is lost? And why should we keep our noses to the grindstone if all work and no play make Jack a dull boy?

Why does the promising stock I buy always plummet the very next day? And why is that drastically reduced designer dress I purchased last week (Final Sale! No Returns!) reduced much further the following week?

How come dedicated vegetarians often wear leather coats,

shoes, and other accessories? Is it okay to kill animals to make us look good but not to nourish us? Maybe they rationalize that since the creature has already been butchered, it's pointless to let its hide go to waste. On the other hand, meat eaters could argue that since a cow has been slaughtered to provide rich Corinthian leather for our furniture and apparel, it would be sinful to toss out those perfectly good T-bones and filet mignons.

How can teenagers understand every word of every rap song when they're completely incomprehensible to the rest of us?

How come everything in my closet shrinks two sizes from one season to the next?

Speaking of clothes, why in the name of Tommy Hilfiger does anyone pay hundreds of dollars for worn, faded jeans with frayed cuffs and holes in the knees? Am I the only one who thinks that those kids who wear the baggy jeans with the crotches down to their knees look ridiculous?

How come the *QE2*, which tips the scale at over 150 tons, can float and I (who weigh considerably less, even after binging on lasagna) can't? Similarly, how can a 400,000-pound 747 stay aloft, yet I drop like a millstone if I stumble on the curb?

And can anyone tell me why it always rains the day after I've washed my car and why my drain backs up the day after my garbage disposal grinds to a halt, necessitating two separate service charges by my plumber?

Also, how come your waiter always pops up to ask, "How is everything?" just as you've stuffed an oversized portion of the entrée into your mouth making an intelligible reply impossible?

And why did the Magi bring gold, frankincense, and myrrh to the baby Jesus? I mean there he was in a stable, lying in a manger. He could have used a comfy bassinette, a cashmere blanket, a couple of sleepers, a carrier seat that could be strapped to the back of the family donkey . . . and I'm sure Mary would have really appreciated a few dozen disposable diapers. I can understand that the scent of frankincense and myrrh might have been welcome, what with all those animals in the stable, but gold? Generous, but a bit impractical—sort of like giving a homeless person a Rolex watch instead of a warm coat and some McDonald's gift certificates. But maybe the Holy Family simply stashed the loot and regifted it the following Christmas.

I've got to stop trying to solve these enigmas and get some sleep. I hate to resort to medication, but I guess I'll take a sleeping pill.

I sure hope it will cause drowsiness.

A Moving Experience

You know how they say we should live every day as if it were our last? Even more important, we should also live every day as if we were moving tomorrow. That would make us think twice about acquiring "stuff." You know, things like that lovely crystal wine decanter (even though you always just pour directly from the bottle); a coffee-bean grinder (that you know in your heart you might use for three days, tops); another food chopper (that you're sure is far superior to the four you already have); a new porcelain figurine (for which you have absolutely no display space); still another pair of shoes (to cram into the closet with the three dozen pairs already jammed in there); ditto more sweaters, shirts, and pants than you can wear in three lifetimes; as well as every new gadget and gizmo that hits the marketplace.

If, like me, you're such an acquirer, it's not surprising that you're also an easy target for every book that promises to help you get organized—which is never going to happen unless you win the lottery and can buy a home with luxuries such as a separate walk-in closet dedicated solely to housing a collection of 150 pairs of stiletto-heeled boots on custom-designed hangers. Not so farfetched. I recently read an article (and saw pictures!) of just such a marvel.

Of course, if you're wealthy enough to afford such fantasies, relocating to a new mansion would be no problem. Your staff would simply arrange to have professional packers and movers come in and take care of it all while you jet off to Bora Bora. (It would be much too traumatic to stick around and watch all those people work. You're not heartless, after all.)

If, however, like me, your budget dictates that you must do all the packing and unpacking yourself, you are so going to regret all those impulsive purchases of the last few years.

I moved a month ago, and I vow never to do anything so rash again. Every step of the operation was a horror—scrounging empty cartons from all the liquor stores and supermarkets in town, spending a fortune on giant rolls of bubble wrap, and swathing every plate, bowl, cup, and mug in the bubble wrap before packing them into the cartons (do you have any idea how time consuming that is?), then stacking the filled cartons on any available floor space.

When I started, I was very efficient, color coding each carton by contents and making a master list. People make too big a deal about moving, I thought. It's a cinch if you're organized. Maybe I'd even write a book about painless moving. I even took time out to craft a rough outline.

By carton twenty-five, I abandoned my system and just starting stuffing items randomly into whatever box had an available few inches of space. As for my master list, I tossed it into the trash, along with my outline for the definitive book about moving efficiently. I also soon ditched my plan to place heavier cartons on the bottom of each pile and started piling large boxes with pots and pans on top of smaller cartons with fragile china. At some point, I even stopped labeling the cartons and had no idea what was in any of them. I toiled for three days, stopping only for calls of nature (thank heaven, I had left a narrow, barely negotiable path to the bathroom).

The stacks grew higher. By the third evening, they began to teeter dangerously. I should do something about that, I thought. Instead, I went to bed. I was exhausted. But who could sleep? I kept expecting to hear the crash of stacks of boxes colliding against each other like falling dominos, knocking down walls and crushing me in my bed.

Actually, that might have been a blessing. It would have spared me the pain of moving into the new place, which turned out to be even more chaotic than the move out of the old. My movers were as inept as I, stacking boxes haphazardly everywhere. Yes, everywhere. Though my new condo has two bathrooms, the paths to both were blocked with cartons by the time they left.

Crying was not an option. I had no idea where my tissues were packed.

I picked a carton at random and opened it. Okay. Some of my china, which belonged in my dining room breakfront—which, of course, was inaccessible. I opened another carton. Pots and pans for the kitchen . . . come on! I knew there was a kitchen here somewhere. I wouldn't have purchased a condo without a kitchen. I put the pots and pans on top of the opened (but still filled) carton with my china. Oh, oh! Did I just hear the sound of shattering crystal?

And so it went. The harder I worked, the bigger the mess I created.

Why did I decide to move? Sure, the old place had no elevator, and my aging knees were not happy climbing three flights of stairs. Yes, I had to share a laundry, and it was down those same three flights of stairs and accessible only from the outside of the building (think icy walk, heavy laundry basket, trick knees . . .). Yes, like me, the complex was aging, and I was concerned about major repairs in the near future ($$$). And yes, it was not connected to the town sewer system and had its own plant that had to be brought up to code every couple of years ($$$$). But I had been there for nine years and had long since found a niche for all my stuff. And even though the new condo was slightly larger and had more closets, I had no idea how it was going to hold all my possessions in all those cartons.

Happy ending: Eventually, I did get everything stowed away, and I disposed of all the empty boxes and acres of bubble wrap (a major accomplishment in itself) and was actually able to see my floors, my own laundry (bliss), my balcony (ditto) . . .

I even found my tissues, but I no longer needed them, except to dab at a few tears of joy.

I marvel at people who move frequently. But maybe it's like childbirth—maybe in time you forget the pain.

I'm not about to test that theory any time soon, however.

But Wait! There's More!

Okay, that's it. My TV has to go. I can't afford to keep it. No, it's not guzzling too much electricity. It's just that every time I turn it on, one of those insidious infomercials is blaring; and unless I'm suddenly struck deaf and blind, odds are it's going to cost me—big time. Sure enough, even though I have vowed countless times never to watch another persuasive product promo, I'm hooked before I can find the channel-changer button on the remote.

For one thing, who can resist that featherweight vacuum cleaner that sucks up everything from a tiny grain of rice to handfuls of Fido's fur embedded in the fibers, with no effort at all on the part of the lovely lass demonstrating the sweeper? Look, she's picking it up with one finger! She's smiling broadly, obviously enjoying herself. I envy her. When was the last time I had fun—and looked gorgeous—while vacuuming? Never, that's when. Hmm . . . maybe I should buy . . .

No! I don't need another vacuum cleaner. I'm changing the channel. But now the sweeper is annihilating a mountain of nuts and bolts. This I have to see. Surely, it will choke on them and die. It doesn't even hiccup.

Could my vacuum do that? I don't know, and why does it matter? I've never spilled a bucket of nuts and bolts on my rugs. I don't have any nuts and bolts in my toolbox. In fact, I don't even own a toolbox. Still, you never know when that might change. It wouldn't hurt to be prepared.

This is getting dangerous. I definitely should switch the channel. Instead, I watch, mesmerized, as the operator presses a button and the handle of the sweeper bends, so she doesn't have to, and glides smoothly under beds, sofas, and even two small children playing on the floor. Oops! They're spilling their gooey, half-melted chocolates all over the rug! Not a problem.

The magic sweeper inhales, and the mess is gone in an instant.

I search frantically for my credit card as I pick up the phone to call the 800 number now flashing on the screen. I have to hurry because if I order within the next twenty minutes, I'll also receive a small cordless hand vacuum cleaner absolutely free of charge! All I will have to pay is additional shipping costs. I hesitate. I'm no dummy. I realize the shipping fee is probably higher than the value of the "free" vacuum.

Feeling very smart, I start to put my credit card away and pick up the remote to turn off the TV—until I hear,

"BUT WAIT! THERE'S MORE!"

If I'm one of the first five hundred people to call, in addition to the magic sweeper and the cordless hand vac, I'll also receive, at no additional charge (except for shipping and handling) not one, but two cordless hand vacs.

"ONE FOR THOSE SMALL SPILLS AT HOME AND ONE FOR YOUR CAR!"

That would be great. My car is such a mess. But I remember my vow not to succumb to TV temptation. I'm not going to do it! It feels good to be strong.

"AND THAT'S NOT ALL!"

The announcer interrupts my self-admiration.

"YOU'LL ALSO RECEIVE—ABSOLUTELY FREE—A TWO-YEAR SUPPLY OF . . ."

I don't even wait to hear the rest before I start dialing. I mean a free two-year supply of anything has to be a deal! That's right, I'm so suckered in, I've forgotten about that shipping fee. Now, where did I put my credit card?

I'm such an easy target. Before I can turn off the TV, another beautiful spokeswoman grabs my attention. She says she's seventy years old. My hearing must really be going. She looks seventeen.

"You heard me!" she says, reading my mind over the airwaves. "And I owe it all to this amazing, priceless beauty cream that eradicates wrinkles and banishes blemishes overnight!"

Unfortunately, the "priceless" beauty cream isn't. Actually, it boasts an astronomical price (plus shipping and handling), but can you really put a price on eternal youth? Besides, you can choose three easy payments. But Wait!! There's More!!! If you pick up your phone and order right now . . .

Okay, so maybe I'm not so naïve as to believe the beauty cream pitch, but what about all those wonderful exercise machines that will give me the body of a supermodel without even breaking a sweat; the fabulous kitchen appliances and cookware that will enable me to prepare gourmet meals fit for royalty before I can say "Rachael Ray"; the keyboard (complete with simple instructions) that will have the Carnegie Hall booking agents knocking down my door; the courses in buying and selling real estate that will bring Donald Trump to his knees, begging me to choose him as my apprentice . . .

They all sound so good. This is bad. I need help. My TV is heavy. I can't toss it out the window by myself.

Who Is Simon?
And What Did He Say?

Whatever happened to the simple play of childhood past?

Today's kids would find our primitive pastimes not only boring, but also pathetically ludicrous—if not incredible.

Did we actually gather outdoors in groups after supper (yes, we had supper—not dinner) every evening to play unsophisticated games like Simon Says, Red Rover, Kick the Can, King of the Hill, and Mother, May I? The last one is especially incongruous. Let's face it. Formally asking Mother's permission to do anything these days is rare—and to incorporate this concept into something we did for fun would seem pretty weird to kids today.

Did we actually play these games on the streets in front of our homes? What about the traffic? Well, as I recall, there was none to speak of. Few people could afford cars. I remember one privileged family down the block bought a brand new Ford. It was gray with maroon fenders. It cost $600! Way beyond the means of the rest of the neighborhood. But it didn't really matter, because back then, most people worked at local businesses and our fathers traveled to their jobs by bus (or on foot, so they could save the ten-cent fare) while our mothers stayed home in their housedresses (yes, housedresses!) and cooked and cleaned all day.

It was a blissfully innocent age. No one worried that while we played outside we might be abducted or caught in the crossfire of warring gangs. We stayed out unsupervised until the streetlights came on (our signal to return home)—skipping rope, or playing tag, hide & seek, crack the whip, stickball, hopscotch . . . running, jumping, climbing . . . constantly on the move. Childhood obesity was rare in that pre-TV/computer/video-game age. A couch potato was a tuber that fell from the bowl on Mom's lap as she peeled while listening to "Stella Dallas," "Backstage Wife," "Our Gal Sunday," or one of her other favorite radio soap operas featuring a plucky woman trying gamely to make her way in a male-dominated world.

Our play was unstructured. No coaches, no practice, no game schedules, no parents on the sidelines yelling encouragement or berating us for our failures. And no fancy equipment or designer-label sportswear and athletic shoes. We had no special sneakers for jogging, walking, biking, or hiking. Our all-purpose Keds served all those functions.

I remember learning to ski. No, not on the slopes of a mountain resort, but on my street, a hill that stayed unplowed all winter. (No traffic, remember?) And no state-of-the-art, expensive gear. My skis were wooden slats, tipped up at the toes, with leather straps that slipped over my everyday rubber galoshes that, in turn, I pulled on over my saddle shoes. No high-tech boots. No clamps. (Come to think of it, all that probably was state of the art at the time.)

Not surprisingly, I suppose, I never became very adept at skiing.

I did learn to roller skate (sort of). No, I didn't have rollerblades. Or shoe skates. My wheels were mounted on two adjustable metal plates that could be shortened or lengthened to fit under my good old saddle shoes; and they attached to my shoes with clamps that were tightened with a roller-skate key. I wore my key on a string around my neck so I wouldn't lose it.

I never did learn to swim, despite the fact that we had relatives who lived by the shore, whom we visited often. It wasn't easy. (No car, remember?). To get there we had to take a bus, then a streetcar (on which I invariably got sick), followed by a ferry, and finally a train. No wonder I couldn't swim. I was probably much too exhausted by the time I got to the beach to do no more than plop on the sand.

I also never had a stuffed animal as a child. Can you believe it? I don't remember feeling deprived, which must mean that none of my friends had any either. Today's kids, on the other hand, can't find their beds (or floors) because they are hidden under mountains of stuffed dolphins, elephants, alligators, turtles, rabbits, ducks, ponies, giraffes, hippos, penguins, whales, dinosaurs, pandas, puppies, kittens, monkeys, lions and tigers and bears—oh, my! And if those aren't enough, they also have clones of all of them that are computer programmable and incorporated into a myriad of electronic games. I have a secret fear that some day all those animal Webkinz are going to band together and take over the world. (Actually, they might do a better job than most of the humans in charge today.)

Though I never had a teddy bear, I wasn't completely toy destitute. I did have a beautiful Shirley Temple doll, AND a baby doll that would drink from a bottle and then wet her diapers! Talk about high tech. I also remember a toy washing machine with a wringer. I know, no one under the age of sixty today remembers washing machines with wringers, but they were really the cat's meow (that's "cool" in today's lingo). Hey, they beat going down to the river and scrubbing your clothes on rocks.

Travel has also evolved exponentially. While today's toddlers jet off to Disney World with their parents while they're still in diapers (the toddlers, not the parents), I took my first flight when I was twenty-five. No—not with the Wright Brothers, but in a propeller-powered plane. Noisy! Slow! Bumpy! But I loved it. I didn't know any better.

Yes, times have changed—and are changing. I can't imagine what the next hundred years will bring. Unfortunately, we won't be here to see. Or maybe we will. I just read that scientists are working on extending the human life span to two hundred and beyond. Apparently, they're not worried about where to put us all. By then, NASA will have established communities on other planets.

I hope there will be plenty of job openings on Venus or Mars or wherever I'm sent, because I'm going to run out of money before I'm one hundred.

Do You Believe That Outfit?

Come on, people! Does anyone really believe that shirttails hanging below sweaters and vests are attractive? When did that look suddenly go from "sloppy" to "chic"?

Apparently, none of the former fashion rules apply. Today you can wear a print blouse with a plaid skirt, an orange jacket with shocking pink pants, a pastel flowered shirt with purple-, green-, and red-striped Capri pants. A recent fashion magazine proclaims "such clashing patterns and colors create a look of carefree spontaneity." Talk about putting a good spin on disaster. What it really says to me is that the wearer got dressed in the dark.

These days, it's a no-no to allow your handbag to harmonize with any element of your outfit. It seems that your purse should make an independent statement of its own.

As for shoes, not only should they not match any other part of your attire, they can also be fabricated from disparate materials of mismatched shades. This is perfectly acceptable, especially if they're expensive enough. In fact, the more costly the footwear, the more outlandish its design. Case in point: I saw an ad today in a slick woman's magazine that featured a $3,000 pair of shoes with black satin toes, brown and tan leather sides, and rhinestone-studded raspberry velvet backs and heels (five-inch stilettos). As if this weren't bad enough, the model wore them with saggy black ankle socks. I swear.

I will say, however, that those socks weren't quite as saggy as the pants favored by young men today. What's with those oversized khakis with the crotches at knee level, the waistband drooping at the hips exposing underpants, and the bottom of the legs draped over unlaced sneakers sweeping the ground? And I never will understand why jeans (both men's and women's) are more expensive if they are already frayed and holey when you buy them.

Women's hemlines are another issue. Can skirts get any shorter? How do you sit without displaying your panties? Many solve this problem simply by not wearing any panties and not worrying about what else may be displayed.

Speaking of immodesty, when did silk and lace camisoles (with adjustable shoulder straps yet) first escape from the underwear drawer and reappear as outerwear for young (and, even more unfortunately, many not so young) women? Not too long ago, we would have been arrested for appearing in public wearing lingerie. Today, it's perfectly acceptable to let it all hang out. And the body parts that are not hanging out are nevertheless clearly visible under fabric so transparent that it leaves nothing to the imagination. Nowadays, one can see on any street or classroom costumes that used to be considered risqué on the burlesque stage.

I know I'm dating myself when I say that when I was a girl we would have died of embarrassment if we thought anyone even suspected we had breasts—and especially nipples. We camouflaged them under baggy sweaters or loose-fitting sack dresses (yes, Dior actually designed such a creation decades ago—and actually called it that—and it actually looked like its name).

Ditto derrières. Our goal was to diminish them—certainly not to call attention to them. The flatter the better. We used to wear girdles to banish our buttocks. Today, instead, the gluteus maximus proudly proclaims its presence under skirts and pants so tight, it's a wonder the wearers can move. And those who haven't been endowed by nature with what they consider enough "junk in the trunk" can buy padded panties to correct the deficiency. Insanity.

I guess it could be worse. At least today's fashions aren't as cumbersome as the togs of some past eras. Consider, for example, those huge stiff ruffled collars worn by the noble ladies of the Elizabethan age. They surely must have immobilized the head, much like the cone apparatus that dogs with eczema have to wear to keep them from biting their sores.

Can you imagine how uncomfortable those dames and duchesses must have been in their multiple floor-length petticoats and restrictive bodices, especially in the heat of summer? Not to mention the outer layers of the garments of both men and women—heavy, unyielding materials such as brocade, damask, or buckram-backed taffeta, depending on one's social status. The more luxurious fabrics could be worn only by the upper crust. By law, the lower classes were restricted to clothing made of wool, linen, or sheepskin—which doesn't sound that bad actually. Fortunately, for the hoi polloi, polyester had not yet been invented; otherwise, I'm sure they would have been doomed to spend their lives encased in nylon.

At least our clothing today is more democratic. We all have the right to look slutty and cheap, regardless of our social standing.

And, of course, the fewer clothes we wear, the easier our laundry. (Wouldn't you have hated to be Elizabeth I's personal maid?)

What's next? Birthday suits as everyday attire? Just in case, I'd better see what I can do to spruce mine up. Right now, it's a wrinkled mess.

Paranoia, Paul Newman, and Other Pet Peeves

I don't care how unflappable you are, I'll bet there are certain things that get your goat, such as expressions like "get your goat." What does that mean? In the first place, how many people actually own a goat? And in the second place, I know if I had one, I'd be delighted to have someone else "get" it, since I understand goats will eat everything in sight, including the door off your refrigerator and your complete Hummel collection. So, yes, meaningless expressions are one of my pet peeves. (And what's with that? If it's a pet, how can it be a peeve?)

Paranoid people also bug me. (How did insects get into this?) You know the type. If you happen to mention something like, "I was reading recently about the destruction of Pompeii . . ." they'll snap back defensively. "I had nothing to do with that! I was in Poughkeepsie that day!"

And speaking of Paul Newman (yes, I was—see title), one of my top peeves for several decades has been that he was never my pet. I always hoped that maybe, one of these days, but now he's gone, and it's too late. Show me where it's written that Joanne Woodward had more right to him all these years than I?

And who is the fiend who designs the layouts for supermarkets? It's no accident that the displays are arranged in such a way that in order to find one lamb chop, a loaf of bread, and a bunch of carrots, you have to weave through all sixteen aisles and nine displays of "specials" you don't need and can't afford but just can't resist (especially if they're fattening). Not only do you spend at least five times the money for ten times the calories you planned, when you get home and unpack all your impulse purchases, you find you've forgotten the carrots.

When I have such a frustrating experience, I try to relax and forget it by going to the movies with a friend. The theater may be completely empty as we sit down. A few seconds later, another couple arrives; and though there are 596 available seats, the only ones that suit them are the two right smack in front of us. It's not easy to love your neighbors when they insist on being that neighborly.

Nor is it easy for me to love women whose hair never frizzes, whose mascara never smears, and who look good in a bikini. Also, women who were married to Paul Newman.

I'm equally annoyed by people who are early when I'm late and late when I'm early. I had several ex-bosses who were very good at this.

Others on my "Unloveables" list are people who feel impelled to forward to me every single e-mail others send to them, regardless of my level of interest in the subject matter. I don't care about the guy who broke the dead-fly-swallowing contest; I am not curious about the mating rituals of the fire ant; and I couldn't care less about how many rifles Charlton Heston collected before he died. Too much information! And I don't want to be promised the fulfillment of my wildest dreams if I forward the e-mail to twenty others—or ten years of bad luck if I don't. Neither do I want to be labeled unpatriotic if I don't forward the latest political propaganda to everyone I've known since kindergarten. I simply want to be able to leave my computer for twenty minutes and not come back to an announcement that I have forty-two new messages (unless at least one of them had been from Paul Newman).

I'm also not too crazy about the genius who first decreed that every garment must be constructed from fabric containing Spandex. If I wanted the world to know about every extra ounce of flab on my body, I would have joined a nudist colony.

And how about the fashion (and philosophy) of today's youth? A recent issue of my alma mater's alumni magazine featured some of the current crop of graduates, including one young lady wearing a flouncy, red/orange/yellow-flowered miniskirt, a black-and-white-striped tee top under a brown sweater, black tights, and army boots. It was no surprise to read that she wants to move to the woods of Maine and live in a tree house for the summer while her roommate (whose costume was equally bizarre) plans to live in a community where she can "grow her own food, make her own furniture and clothes, and develop personal bartering and trade relationships." For this, they needed a college education?

Then there are those friends I travel with who insist on getting to the airport four hours before flight time . . . and those who aren't happy unless we manage to get through security just as they're disconnecting the Jet way from the plane prior to takeoff.

Speaking of travel, passports should not be issued to people like the American tourist I met on one of my trips who loudly complained that the ice cream on the Via Veneto isn't like Schrafft's or that some "stupid foreigner" whom he stopped for directions couldn't speak English, even though the "foreigner" (who was in his native country) could probably speak four or five other languages, and the American's linguistic ability extended only to third-grade English and basic pig Latin.

I also have a beef (first insects—now cows?) with ads that feature the phrase, "For your convenience." Whatever they're offering, you can be sure that it's not for your convenience; it's for their profit.

That's almost, but not quite, as bad as the phone message that tells you, "Your call is important to us" before you are put on hold until sunset—or sunrise, whichever comes last.

Then there's the guy who knows everything, and what he doesn't know, he'll fake. He also claims to be able to do anything better than anyone else. You tell him the latest world record in any field (be it alligator wrestling, sky diving, tiddlywinks, whatever), and he'll tell you he topped it at least a year ago. Ten to one he'll maneuver you into a corner at a cocktail party and proceed to deliver a monotonous monologue describing every meaningless moment of his oh, so dull life, starting with his toilet training at four months old (the youngest on record). It's agonizing. All those times I was forced to listen to him, I couldn't mingle with the other guests. (Paul Newman could have been in the other room, for all I knew.)

But enough of this. If I don't stop, you're going to think I'm a chronic complainer—and I hate chronic complainers. They're one of my pet peeves.

Too Much of a Good Thing

Many people believe that too much of a good thing is wonderful. I'm not one of them.

Take shoes, for instance. Like most women, I love them. But enough already! When I was a child, I had three pairs of shoes: One for school (penny loafers or saddle shoes), one for play (Keds), and one for Sundays (black-patent Mary Janes). Today, I'm embarrassed to admit, I have more than three dozen pairs. A ridiculous waste. Not only of money, but also of valuable time. Every morning, I spend at least five minutes trying to decide which shoes to wear—and nine times out of ten, I simply don the ones I wore the day before. I'm retired. I don't have to impress anyone, so what does it matter? Later, if I decide to get some exercise, I have to choose among several pairs of sneakers, some with designer logos (again, I'm ashamed to confess), depending on whether I plan to hike, jog, use my stationary bike, or simply take a leisurely walk; because nowadays, each activity requires different footwear. At least that's what "they" tell us. And we listen. How crazy is that?

Then there's the whole question of what to put on the rest of my body. My three spacious closets are jammed with pants, skirts, sweaters, shirts, and dresses—many of which I haven't worn in a decade. Others still have price tags from stores that went out of business five years ago. Apparently, they lost their appeal on the trip from the shops to home. Why am I keeping them?

If I cleared my closets of all that extraneous stuff, I'd finally have someplace to put my vacuum cleaner. Maybe all three of them, in fact. Come to think of it, I haven't a clue as to why I have three vacuum cleaners. I seldom use any of them (another embarrassing revelation).

It seems no one believes that less is more. Take automobiles, for instance. When I was a kid (yes, we did have cars then!), it was easy to identify a Ford, a Chevrolet, a Chrysler. No longer. Not only because dozens of foreign cars are also rolling off the assembly lines onto traffic-choked American highways, but also because every manufacturer turns out dozens of models that all look like clones of each other. Not a distinctive design in the bunch.

Shopping for anything is a challenge these days—be it cars, computers, cameras, calculators, cosmetics, cornflakes, cookies (and many other products starting with "C," plus the other twenty-five letters of the alphabet). So many brands. So many claims. So many prices. By the time you finish evaluating all your options, they are obsolete, only to be replaced by an even more confusing assortment.

Meanwhile, meals (in restaurants and most homes) have exploded to supersized portions—as have candy bars, popcorn buckets, and "big gulp" soft drinks at movie theaters. The theaters themselves have evolved from the one-screen movie houses of my youth to today's multiplexes offering a choice of twenty or more films.

Excess rules everything these days, including TV. One twelve-inch, fuzzy black-and-white set used to be enough for the entire family. Now sixty+-inch plasmas in high-definition color are sprouting in every living room, den, bedroom, playroom, kitchen, patio, and even some bathrooms. Furthermore, I can remember when we had only three network channels. To be truthful, I can even remember BTV (before television), when radio was our only in-home entertainment. Today, cable TV offers us hundreds of channels. It's overwhelming. We can watch only one at a time. But since TiVo enables us to record many others, we soon accumulate a huge backlog of programs that we'll never find time to watch because we're too busy checking the dozens of e-mails that pop up on our computers hourly and ridding our mailboxes of hunks of junk, including all those mail-order catalogs I receive every day.

Many moons ago I made the mistake of ordering a couple of items from catalogs, which I now realize was a big mistake because apparently my name and address were distributed to every mail-order company in the country—and several overseas—who keep deluging me with their glossy publications, which I don't even open. They go directly from my mailbox to my recycle bin. Think of the wasted printing costs and postage, to say nothing of the poor mailman's aching back. More important, it saddens me to think of how many rainforests are being destroyed to supply the paper for all those annoying, unread, unwanted mailings.

Speaking of which, I've completely lost patience with all those charity solicitations enclosing sheets of return-address mailing labels, which are meant to guilt me into sending a donation. News flash! It doesn't work. At least not with me. In fact, these "gift" labels turn me off whichever charity sends them to me. I have accumulated more than I'll ever need. If they keep coming, I swear I'll move and not leave a forwarding address. And if that doesn't work, maybe I can talk myself into the witness protection program and disappear to an undisclosed location where the junk mailers won't be able to find me.

And what about all those electronic gadgets that we used to get along without but that have now become necessities of life—cell phones, Blackberries, GPS devices, digital cameras whose inch-square memory cards hold hundreds of images, and tiny iPods on which you can download thousands of songs (or the noise that passes for music today).

Dealing with all these excesses is exhausting and time consuming. But maybe that's a good thing. After all, doctors say that keeping busy is the key to longevity.

If that's true, at this rate I should live to at least 220, especially with the help of the countless vitamin supplements and prescription medication available these days. The only problem is that you're supposed to "call your doctor" before taking them. If we all did that, doctors would have time to do nothing but answer their phones 24/7.

The last time I tried to call mine, I learned that she had joined the newly formed PPP (Physicians Protection Program) and had moved to an undisclosed location.

Where Have They Gone?

Do you ever wonder where all the secretaries of the world have gone? They used to be ubiquitous in the old days. Business could not be conducted without them. For a while, they were replaced by "executive assistants" (actually, just another name for secretaries—same duties, but a fancy title instead of a raise). Today's executives don't need assistants, at least not to type their letters. They do that themselves on computers. Yep, typewriters have also disappeared. Come to think of it, letters (the old-fashioned kind printed on paper and mailed in envelopes) are also becoming obsolete. "Snail mail" is out. E-mail rules.

It also occurs to me that the secretaries have not gone alone into Never-Never Land. With them are all the blushing virgin brides of yesteryear. One of the advantages of the disappearance of that antiquated concept is that a couple's children can now attend their parents' wedding. Premarital pregnancies used to be considered shameful. Today, they're celebrated, with celebrities leading the way. Open any issue of *People* magazine, for example, and you'll see photos of unwed starlets proudly displaying their "baby bumps" and accepting congratulations from one and all.

And when/if a couple do get married, should the promise to "forsake all others as long as you both shall live" still be part of the vows? It seems to me that it's no longer a question of if that pledge will be kept but, rather, how soon it will be broken.

Remember the milkman who used to deposit your daily dairy

supply on your back stoop, probably while the Fuller Brush man was ringing your front doorbell? (Come to think of it, how did the Fuller Brush man manage to make a living? How many brushes does anyone need?)

Then there was the door-to-door encyclopedia salesman. Every family's goal was to own an entire Britannica set to give their children a leg up with their schoolwork. Today, Wikipedia tells us everything Britannica ever did and so much more—and, unlike the encyclopedia contents, all that Wikipedia data is always up-to-the-minute.

Also disappearing are road maps, which are being replaced by GPS devices featuring a friendly voice that leads you, turn by turn, to your destination. However, if you don't pay attention and make a wrong turn, the voice becomes less friendly and orders you to "make a legal U-turn when possible!" But that's nowhere near as annoying as having to refold a road map.

And where has modesty gone? The woman who is not displaying at least four inches of cleavage (and no panty lines because she's not wearing panties) is definitely overdressed; and bodies not decorated with tattoos and multiple piercings are becoming rarer every day.

Speaking of wearing apparel, when was the last time you saw a housedress or an apron? Or a woman's hat? No, not a visored cap—a real hat with flowers, feathers, a veil . . .

These days, pay phones and phone booths are almost obsolete because of the proliferation of cell phones. I worry about where Clark Kent can change into his Superman suit.

And why do we still talk about dialing numbers on a phone when we push buttons instead?

Also gone are the old mom-and-pop grocery stores, along with their nonautomated cash registers. Mom and Pop actually had to do real math to add up the total cost of the groceries you bought and figure out how to give you change from a ten-dollar bill. (Yes, you actually could buy a week's worth of groceries for less than ten dollars in the olden days.) Today's kids who work in modern supermarkets would be stymied if the power went out just after the computerized register said you owe $99.98. Hand them $100, and they would have no idea how much change to give you.

Are you old enough to remember when gas stations were called "service stations"? Do you know why? Because you actually got service there. A smiling attendant would not only pump your gas, he'd clean your windshield, check your oil and water, and even kick your tires if you asked him to.

Kitchens aren't what they used to be either—thank God. They now have dishwashers (not the lady of the house, but an automatic appliance), stoves with self-cleaning ovens, refrigerators instead of iceboxes, and counters that hold a variety of electric devices that mix, purée, chop, grate, peel, core, and cook entire meals with minimal help from a human. And they do all that while a robot vacuum cleaner sucks up the dirt from all the carpeting in the rest of your house. All you have to do is press a button.

Unfortunately, I still have to clean my own toilets. Despite all the products available to make the job easier, I still have to apply some elbow grease to the brush. I haven't found a robot yet that will go into the bowl and do it for me.

And what has happened to the bar soaps we used to have in our bathrooms and kitchens. Now our soap comes in bottles. I never saw that coming.

In restaurants (and in most homes) normal portions have given way to supersized meals and snacks (how do you spell F-A-T). On airplanes, on the other hand, food has all but disappeared. They may still serve meals in first class, but how would I know?

Does anyone still have a TV with rabbit ears or a rooftop antenna? Does any home still have a coal bin? One of my early family homes had one (I'm really showing my age here); but before we moved out, my parents had installed an oil burner and cleaned and painted the coal bin and converted it to a basement bar. I'll drink to that. Except I couldn't then. I was too young.

Also on the endangered species list are film and the cameras that use it. Can't say I miss them. I remember toting a bulky Kodak Instamatic, several cartons of flashbulbs, and three dozen rolls of film on my first trip to Europe, constantly worrying about keeping track of all the film and protecting it from the radiation of airport security checks. There were a lot of those, since I was on a ten-countries-in-fourteen-days trip. I was also very concerned about whether I was getting any good shots. With my tiny digital camera (with built-in flash), a postage-stamp-size memory card takes a few hundred pictures. What's more, I can instantly see the results of each effort and retake the unsatisfactory ones. I would have enjoyed my early travels so much more if digital cameras had been available decades ago.

I could go on and on. But I do have other things to do—like laundry. I have to traipse down to the cellar and get out the washtub and scrub board. . . . No! I forgot! I have a washer and dryer now!

Progress. It's wonderful. Even if virgin brides had to be sacrificed to achieve it.

What Does It Really Mean?

Have you ever stopped to analyze the real meaning of all those phrases that we're bombarded with daily by people who are trying to sell us something?

For example, "One size fits all" means that it doesn't fit anyone correctly. Trust me. It's going to be either too loose or too tight, too short or too long.

"For your convenience . . ." has nothing whatsoever to do with your convenience. It's for their profit and/or benefit.

"Thank you for your patience!" is a phrase usually heard when you've been on hold for ten minutes or more, subjected to music you would never have selected if you had a choice. Who's been patient?! If they had been listening, they would have heard you cursing and fuming.

"Ask your doctor," means, "Buy this drug. It's ridiculously overpriced, and one of the dozens of possible serious side effects is death; but we want your money." They know you're not really going to "ask your doctor" who, you can be sure, is not waiting by the phone for your call.

Moreover, don't you love the old, "Thank you for calling XYZ Company." You have a complaint about their product; or maybe they haven't sent the rebate they promised; or they charged more than the advertised price. Who else would you call?

A warning: Whenever you hear "To thank you for your order, we'd like to offer you the opportunity to . . .," hang up immediately and run for the hills! The only opportunity they're offering you is the "privilege" of buying a ridiculously expensive product or service that you don't need, don't want, and can't afford. Often, for example, you will be offered a free copy of a few magazines, which "you may enjoy at no charge." Yes, that's true. But by accepting, you're automatically locked into subscribing to the magazines. Of course, if you want to discontinue the subscriptions, all you have to do is write "cancel" on their invoice when you receive it. There's the catch. You probably won't get an invoice for several weeks, by which time you will automatically pay it because you will have forgotten your option to cancel and will simply assume you must have legitimately subscribed.

Also, beware of those "limited time only!" inducements, and sales pitches that urge you to "be one of the first one hundred callers" in order to receive a special reduced price. Just for fun, I've tried calling some of those numbers six months after the fact, and I still hear, "Congratulations! You are one of the first one hundred callers, so by ordering today, you are eligible for a 50 percent discount!" If they really haven't had more than one hundred calls in six months, how come they're still in business?

As a rule, whenever you hear or read the word "congratulations!" in a sales pitch, you can be sure it's not good news. Almost as dangerous are the words "You have been chosen to receive," which translate to "Welcome to our sucker list."

Then there's one of my favorites: "Your call is important to us." Yeah, right. That's why they'll leave me hanging on hold for thirty minutes.

And how many people are taken in by the offer of a free sample of anything? "All you pay are the shipping and handling costs!" which generally total much more than the value of the sample.

When will we finally learn not to be taken in by offers that sound too good to be true? Log on to the Internet, and a flashing message tells you, "You have just won a free laptop! Click here to claim your prize!" Open your mail and out tumbles a card with instructions to scratch some circles and match the winning number to win a free vacation! (Amazingly, you always match the winning number.) Answer your telephone, and a breathless voice tells you that you are eligible to receive a free car! Sure, and the first Sunday of November will fall on a Tuesday this year. None of it is real. There is always a costly catch.

What about those free, no-obligation trials? Are you really going to go through the trouble (and considerable expense) of returning that treadmill, forty-two-inch LCD TV, computer desk, or whatever heavy, cumbersome contraption you ordered in a moment of weakness?

Disturbing as all this is, however, the three words that strike the most terror in my heart are "some assembly required." Last week, for example, I made the mistake of flipping through one of the many catalogs that clog my mailbox regularly, and I ordered what appeared to be a simple, small end table, even though the ad included the dreaded "some assembly required" caveat. A couple of weeks later, a huge carton arrived containing a rainforest's worth of paper packing material, a dozen wooden components, and approximately ninety-five nuts, bolts, screws, and other unidentifiable gizmos. I knew I could never assemble it because I don't have an engineering degree from MIT. My neighbor does; so I knocked on his door, and he generously offered his services. However, after two unsuccessful hours, he was reduced to a quivering mass of insecurity. He mumbled an apology, threw everything back into the carton, and fled to enroll in graduate school.

By the way, I still have that carton of components in the back of my closet.

Congratulations! Just send me your name and address, and I will be happy to send it to you, absolutely free! All you need pay are shipping and handling costs.

Self-Improvement or Self-Delusion?

I don't understand it. How come I don't have flat abs, buns of steel, and firm thighs and upper arms?

I have shelled out big bucks for every available exercise video targeting those areas, at least a dozen books illustrating ways to achieve those goals, as well as a treadmill, an exercise bike, a rowing machine, and—most recently—an exercise ball. I even bought a gorgeous designer jogging suit and one-hundred-dollar sneakers. But no results.

I probably do have flat abs, but they're still buried under layers of flab; my buns are still more Entenmann's than steel; and my thighs and upper arms still have the consistency of unset Jell-O.

So why am I not in shape? My doctor tells me that good intentions and maxing out my credit cards for the videos and exercise equipment and books don't do the job. She claims that I have to *use* the equipment I bought and actually *do* the exercises demonstrated in the videos and books. Is that true?

I also invested in at least a dozen diet books—Atkins, Pritikin, the Zone, South Beach . . . Do you suppose the reason they didn't work was because the only one I in fact tried was *The Nine-Day Ice Cream Diet?* Maybe I should have guessed that that one belongs in the "if it sounds too good to be true" category.

I also have similar problems in other areas of my life. Take digital photography, for example. I bought a state-of-the art camera. Too many bells and whistles. I couldn't figure out how to use the blasted thing. Forget the manual that came with it. Like most computer-related instructions, it was written by a techie who assumes that the average layperson graduated from MIT, summa cum laude.

The same with housework. I have spent a ton of money on every new miracle mop, magnetic duster, and magical cleaning potion to hit the supermarket shelves and be featured in TV infomercials. Somehow, I never seem to have the time to use them. I'm much too busy avoiding exercise, buying more diet books while making excuses not to diet, and writing complaint letters to the manufacturer of my digital camera.

I did buy a robot vacuum cleaner so I could at least have clean carpets without any effort on my part. Unfortunately, I have yet to learn how to use the remote to keep it from choking on the fringe of scatter rugs or getting stuck under furniture and frantically beeping for me to come and rescue it. What's more, I discovered it expects me to empty its dustbin from time to time. For what it cost, shouldn't it be smart enough to open the door, go outside, and throw up its contents without any help from me?

Also, considering how many foreign-language learning tools— books, videos, and courses (both on site and online)—I've bought over the past several years, I should easily be able to dash off this essay in Italian and French, as well as English, and thereby broaden my market exponentially.

Unfortunately, again, I eventually realized that the amount of money spent on instructional resources does not translate into results. The hidden requirement of expending effort, as well as $$$, is always there. It doesn't seem fair somehow.

On second thought, maybe that's a good thing. It's comforting to know that the rich do not have an advantage over the rest of us when it comes to self-improvement. Or do they?

Yeah, actually they do.

Take exercise, for instance. Sure, even the wealthy have to work out to achieve results; but they can afford to have a personal trainer to motivate them in their own modern home gyms, and they can swim laps in their indoor and outdoor Olympic-sized pools. Or they can forego the physical effort completely and simply pay an eminent liposuction specialist top dollar to suction the fat out of their problem areas.

As for dieting, somehow I think it must be a lot easier when you have your own in-house chef (a Cordon Bleu graduate with a master's degree in nutrition) creating low fat, but yummy repasts and snacks.

The same applies to educational pursuits. If I didn't have to wade through all the indecipherable manuals and could instead afford to hire a Bill Gates wannabe to give me one-on-one lessons on my digital camera, computer, whatever, I, too, could become a technical guru. As for learning a foreign language, spending quality time cavorting with the natives in Paris and Rome would be tons more fun and a lot more productive than trying to memorize irregular verb conjugations from books and tapes.

And while I am "studying" with François and Giovanni, a staff of servants would keep my estate spotless, with absolutely no sweat off my brow.

Unfortunately, until I win the lottery, none of that is going to happen for me. If I want to change my life, I'm just going to have to apply myself and become more disciplined. But how?

Wait. I just remembered. Yesterday I saw an ad for a book titled *A Sure-Fire Formula for Self-Motivation.* Just what I need. I must run out and buy it immediately.

I know it will work—if I can figure out how to motivate myself to read it.

What Will They Think of Next?

There's nothing new under the sun.

That may have been true centuries ago when the phrase was attributed to an unnamed philosopher, identified only as "the Preacher," in the Book of Ecclesiastes; but since then, WOW! Innovations have been flying at us at the speed of light.

Every time I think things have gone as far as they can, I remember the song from the Rodgers and Hammerstein musical "Oklahoma" that proclaimed, "Everything's up to date in Kansas City."

"I counted twenty gas buggies goin' by theirselves, almost every time I took a walk," the singer reports, "An' then I put my ear to a Bell telephone, an' a strange woman started into talk . . . they've gone about as 'fer' as they can go."

Hardly. Obviously, they've gone a heck of a lot "ferer." Some "buggies" no longer need gas. They run on electricity. And no woman, strange or otherwise, talks to you when you pick up a telephone, Bell or otherwise. At least not a live one. Most likely, you'll hear a recorded voice—not necessarily female. And that phone probably doesn't even have a wire; but it does play music and take pictures, and has a global positioning satellite system and Internet access—and, who knows, soon maybe the ability to sprout wings and fly you to Mars.

The song continues, "They went an' built a skyscraper seven stories high, about as high as a buildin' otta grow."

Of course, today's skyscrapers actually do scrape the sky,

while back in the Kansas City of yore, "With every kind of comfort every house is all complete. You can walk to privies in the rain and never wet your feet! They've gone about as fer as they can go."

Not quite. Indoor privies have since morphed into luxury spas, with giant Jacuzzis, tanning beds, toilets that flush automatically, and showers for two (or more) with dozens of power jets.

All well and good, but I wish the brainiacs who developed these wonders would turn their attention to more practical areas—like designing a fitted sheet that will fold itself. I still haven't figured out how to do it manually.

Also, how about a shopping cart that will survey your fridge and pantry, print out a shopping list of what you need, and maybe even roll itself to the supermarket to collect your groceries. Okay, so that may be a bit unreasonable. Actually, I'd settle for a cart whose wheels all go in the same direction.

I'd really appreciate a dishwasher that loads and unloads itself and stows all the clean dishes, glasses, flatware, and pots and pans in their designated places. Again, if that's too much to ask, how about one that actually delivers on its promise to clean those pots and pans of burnt-on food without any help from me?

I do have a robotic vacuum cleaner, but I don't know why. I don't really trust it, so I go over all the rugs with my electric manual vac anyway. And I still have to dust. Will someone please design a feather duster that can flutter around on its own, cleaning every surface, nook and cranny, including the ones I usually miss?

Oh, and you know what else would be great—house plants with feet that could walk over to the kitchen sink and water themselves when they're thirsty. All that droopy, dried foliage perched on various surfaces in my home does nothing to enhance its décor.

Sure, they've invented a car that can parallel park itself, but when will they give us one that will drive itself down the highway so I can concentrate on my cell phone calls, answer my e-mail on my laptop, and use both hands to eat my sandwich without worrying that a cop is going to pull me over.

Also on my wish list (actually at the top) is a magic wand that I can wave over my lasagna and hot fudge sundae to absorb all the calories. In the meantime, I'd like a scale that will lie and tell me I've finally lost those twenty pounds. And until someone develops a wrinkle cream that really works, how about a mirror that lies, too?

I'd also really appreciate drawers and cupboards that organize themselves, and closets that vaporize anything I haven't worn in two years.

And is there a botanist out there who can develop grass that grows only a couple of inches high and never needs mowing or watering but stays lush and green all summer? Oh, what the heck, all winter, too, while we're at it.

Speaking of winter, will some climatologist please find a way to direct all snow only to the mountains to keep the skiers happy, and off the walks and roadways to keep me happy?

The pundits say that a sure way to wealth is to find a need and fill it. There you go! I've identified many needs. The rest is up to you.

I'll trust you to split the profits with me when they start rolling in.

The Holiday Hustle Hassle

I still remember how I used to love Christmas. That's really amazing considering how bad my memory is and how long it's been since the sight of tinsel and holly and the sound of "Jingle Bells" have made me joyous instead of nauseous.

Looking back, I think the magic disappeared just about the time the big kids told me there was no Santa Claus. Even at that tender age, my precocious little mind must have deduced that if Santa didn't bring all those swell presents, someone sure as heck had to go out and buy them. Goodbye Ho, Ho, Ho! Hello, Boo Hoo, Hoo!

Since then, Christmas shopping has become my second least favorite activity (the first is having a root canal); and it gets progressively worse each year as it becomes increasingly harder to figure out what to buy people that they would like and haven't already bought a more expensive version of for themselves. This is a pretty revealing indication of how paradoxical our society is. Though everyone complains about how tough it is to make ends meet, most of the complaining seems to be done either behind the wheel of one of the two (or more) family cars or in front of the sixty-inch LCD TV and usually by people who have a weight problem caused by an overabundance of rich food and drink.

Years ago, when we "poor" people really had it rough, gift selection was no problem. Aunt Clara was delighted if you bought her a pair of silk (does anyone remember silk?) stockings. (Does anyone remember stockings? They were like pantyhose, only

161

split in half and without the panty). Of course, if she preferred panties, you bought her a pair of "snuggies."

These were like bikini underpants, except they were knee length, high waisted, and made of flannel. And Uncle Joe was happy with a couple of handkerchiefs. These were something like Kleenex, only they were fabric (usually cotton, which you'll remember if you remember silk), and you washed and reused them instead of throwing them away.

As for the children, we've all heard stories from the old folks of how they used to be beside themselves with joy if they found so much as an orange, instead of a lump of coal, in their Christmas stockings. Today, it's not so easy to please a kid. Unless the eight-foot tree is completely hidden behind a pile of bionic, electronic, computerized, overautomated, and overpriced toys that cost more than you used to have to spend to furnish an entire house (real, not doll), they start reading you their Constitutional rights. (They interpret the dictum that "all men are created equal" to mean they should get as many expensive presents as the spoiled rich brat across town.)

Yep, things sure have changed. The only way an orange would please a child today would be if he got to pick it himself from a tree growing in Disneyland.

And, as I said, every year it gets worse—and it starts earlier. The Christmas ads (which used to be respectful enough to wait until the Thanksgiving turkey was cold) now compete for space with ads for the post-Fourth-of-July sales (which start appearing in May). I speak the truth. I swear that last June, the local Holiday Inn's marquee proclaimed, RESERVE NOW FOR CHRISTMAS PARTIES. I wanted to throw up. Instead, I started my Christmas shopping and really got ill. Not that Macy's and Nordstrom aren't lovely stores, but they weren't where I had planned to spend my summer vacation—or the money I had saved up for my summer vacation.

You would not believe the problems I had. Aunt Clara is now out of snuggies (which used to cost $1.98) and into designer tennis dresses (which cost $300), and her thighs looked much better in the snuggies. Uncle Joe has given up handkerchiefs and developed a hankering for Tommy Hilfiger. No, Uncle Joe has not turned gay; he just likes Tommy's expensive jeans, which he mistakenly believes make him look young and hip.

As for the kids on my list, all the little boys already own everything from mini sports cars (guaranteed not to exceed thirty miles per hour for safety reasons) to backyard tree houses with indoor plumbing. And the girls are all flying to Paris with their parents regularly to replenish their Barbie dolls' wardrobes at Christian Dior. Now I ask you, what in the name of Rudolph do you buy these little sophisticates to put the old Christmas sparkle in their eyes?

Selecting gifts for my friends was no easier. It seems we keep playing, "Can you top this?" You know how it is. If you think Richard is going to squander fifty bucks on you, you feel you must spend at least sixty dollars for something he probably will never wear, eat, display, or splash on his face or body. The choice of gift isn't important. The main concern is that it be in the right price range, which escalates every year.

Where is it going to end? Probably in the poor house. Except, come to think of it, poor houses no longer exist. The people who used to go there are now on welfare and living better than you and I. And they have the added advantage that no one expects any holiday presents from them. After all, they're on welfare. And with the price of postage these days, no one even expects them to send Christmas cards.

This brings me to my third least favorite activity—sending Christmas cards. I hate buying them, I hate paying the postage to mail them, and I really hate addressing them. More than that, I hate trying to decide who to send them to. Every year I go through the same weed-out-the-list exercise. I tell myself it's silly to send cards to people I see regularly since I can wish them a happy holiday in person. So I scratch these friends from the list—until

I receive cards from them, at which point they go right back on. Stupid, huh? But what's even dumber is leaving on the list the people I never see and hardly ever hear from. The so-called logic behind this goes something like this: Gee, I haven't seen or spoken to the Smiths for twenty years, and the only time we touch base is at Christmas, so I really should send a card. Why? After two decades of not communicating except for holiday cards, we no longer have anything in common. There might be more point to it, if we at least exchanged letters at Christmas (and I *don't* mean those boastful, Xeroxed lies), but we don't. They send me a card, usually with just a printed greeting and name, and I send them one that I at least sign myself. And to make it more personal, I also usually add a terribly original phrase such as, "Have a great holiday!" And we forget each other for another year. Is this keeping in touch? Since I no longer keep a list of people who send me cards, I have a terrible feeling that, unbeknownst to me, half the people on my list may be dead—and I'm still sending them cards. I hope at least that they're being forwarded.

All of which goes to explain why Christmas makes me nauseous. But from now on, it's going to be different! No more expensive gifts! No more cards to the world at large! Come January 1, I'm making a New Year's resolution—which reminds me of my fourth least favorite activity. But that's a whole other story.

Those Lucky Kids

It's funny. Kids can't wait to grow up so they can enjoy adult privileges. What they don't realize is that, in return, they'll have to give up more than they'll gain. Think of all the things those lucky kids can do that a grown-up can't.

Today, for instance, I saw a little girl wearing a genuine imitation Indian chief's headdress, skipping rope on her front walk. She seemed to be having such a good time that I had a wild urge to buy a feathered war bonnet and a jump rope and go home and do the same thing. But I squashed it. I didn't think I'd enjoy the part when they took me away in a straitjacket.

And that's not the only thing a kid can do that an adult can't. A kid can play house without having to worry about paying off the mortgage.

All a little kid has to do to have everyone think he's a genius is to learn to tie his own shoelaces—or use the potty. Think about it. When was the last time you were applauded for doing that?

A kid looks cute even with two front teeth missing. And every time he loses a tooth, he gets money from the good fairy. And before long, he even gets a replacement tooth, without the expense and pain of an implant.

A kid can ride a skateboard. A grown-up can, too, of course; but he'd have to keep the cast on longer.

A kid can slop paint indiscriminately all over a piece of paper, and Mom will praise it enthusiastically and immediately put it on display on the fridge. Come to think of it, Jackson Pollock did the same thing, but his paintings are too big for the fridge.

A kid can feel insecure without having all his friends recommend a marvelous psychiatrist. And if he feels insecure enough, he can sit right down and cry, no matter where he is. You try that and see what happens.

A kid can go on a candy binge, and the worst he'll suffer is a brief tummy ache. No morning-after problems for him.

A little girl can play with her dolls until she gets tired of them; and she doesn't have to feed them, sing them to sleep, or hire a babysitter when she goes out.

No matter where he goes, even if he doesn't speak the language—or any language, if he's too young—a kid can always find another kid to play with. And he doesn't care what color the other kid's skin is or what house of worship he attends.

A kid can eat cotton candy while riding the merry-go-round without looking foolish.

No one looks at a little blonde girl and wonders if her hair color came from a bottle. She can wear a topless bathing suit on any beach at all, or even her front yard, without being arrested.

A kid can go to the movies—or around the world—for half price. Actually, so can a senior citizen; but the kid doesn't have to take a hearing aid and arthritis pills with him.

He can even get away with pulling a puppy's tail without having the puppy snap at him—or pulling off Grammy's wig without having Grammy snap at him.

If a kid tries to put a round peg in a square hole, no one thinks he's crazy. They just admire his determination.

It's not all roses, of course. A kid does have to worry about arithmetic and scoring a goal at the soccer game to make Mom and Dad proud. On the other hand, he doesn't have to worry about crabgrass, income tax, the checking account balance, social security, or falling hair.

A kid can tell his best friend off and still be his best friend the next day.

When a kid goes to the doctor for a shot, he gets a lollipop if he doesn't cry. A grown-up doesn't cry (at least he'd better not), but all he gets is the bill. Then he might cry a little.

A kid can play baseball during football season and wear his football helmet to the beach in July, and no one thinks it's strange.

A kid can believe in Santa Claus, or at least pretend to—which pays off just as well. And a kid doesn't have to wait for Christmas. He can get almost anything he wants just by promising not to bite the dentist on his next visit.

A kid can sleep in a bunk bed.

A kid has top priority in talking to God.

In fact, a kid has so much going for him, I almost hate him— except I feel sorry for him because he's going to grow up some day and become an adult.

The poor kid.

Can You Hear Me Now?

"I just got on the train, and I couldn't wait to tell you," he shrieked into his cell phone while stowing his duffel bag in the overhead rack. "Guess who knocked on my door last night? That's right! No, I'm not kidding! She said she's thrilled that I moved into the building! And get this—she was wearing skintight short shorts and a tank top with a neckline down to her belly button, which was pierced, by the way! Her tongue, too! She invited me down for a drink when I get back! I tell you, she's hot to trot!" (The guy spoke only in exclamatory clichés.)

I shot a dirty look across the aisle. I wondered if he was oblivious to the fact that he was sharing his news flash not only with his friend on the wireless connection, but also with everyone else within earshot—half the car, at least. Since he was speaking so loudly, I decided he was very aware of his broadcast range and was obviously trying to impress all his fellow passengers either about his upcoming sexual exploits with his new neighbor or merely that he had a cell phone.

If the latter, it didn't work because, unfortunately, he wasn't the only one. As they settled into their seats, dozens of other riders pulled out their own phones and shared with the rest of us details (some embarrassingly intimate, some incredibly boring) of their personal lives. Fragments of conversation assaulted me from all directions:

"It was the worst dental experience I ever had! Five shots of

Novocain, and the pain was still excruciating. The SOB was leaning so hard on the damn drill, I expected him to strike oil any minute!"

"I miss you too, sweetie. . . . No! I miss you more. . . . It seems more like two years, not just two hours. . . . I love you. . . . No, I love you more. . . . Yes, I do. . . . No, you hang up first. . . . No, you."

". . . so I'm selling the whole effing portfolio . . . I'm sick of this whole effing market . . . and that goes for the effing company, too. I'm gonna unload it and spend the winters in Tahiti and summers at my Lake Como villa. . . . No, I've had it with effing Gstaad. That effing chalet has been nothing but trouble since I bought it."

"Hey, Joe. It's me. Thanks for getting me to the station on time. I just barely made it. So what's new?" (Wait a minute. Didn't he just drop you off? What could be new since then?)

When Alexander Graham Bell spoke those innocuous words, "Mr. Watson, come here. I want you," into his "electrical speech machine" in 1876, I'm sure he had no idea that his invention would spawn a cellular monster.

What did people do before cell phones? Actually, we managed to function perfectly well. In fact, it was wonderful. No matter how much our home lives were interrupted by the ringing of the telephone, at least when we were on the road, the rails, or in the air, we could always count on a peaceful respite. We'd be out of touch. No one could reach us. Bliss. But the party's over. Today, hardly anyone leaves home without a cell phone.

At first, a select affluent few had car phones. I envied them so. How comforting it would be not to have to worry about getting a flat tire on a deserted road late at night. Later, phones began to appear on airplanes. A boon for passengers who wanted to notify a loved one or a business associate that their flight was delayed. A great idea, I thought.

But seemingly overnight, the cellular craze mushroomed. Still, the beast might have been somewhat controlled; then the worst happened: Unlimited calling plans were introduced, giving users free rein to give voice to every inconsequential thought, every trivial detail.

Consequently, almost every driver you see has one hand on the steering wheel and the other clutching a cell phone. Either that or they're talking into unseen microphones, making it look as though they're babbling to themselves while hurtling down the highway. It's very disconcerting.

Not just travelers have a wireless umbilical cord to the world. So does every jogger in the park ("I just completed mile five; I should be home in half an hour; on second thought, I'd better slow it down from here, so I'll see you in about forty minutes."); every shopper in the supermarket ("Honey, they don't have super crunchy peanut butter; shall I just get crunchy?"); every sunbather on the beach ("I'm gonna catch a few more rays . . . can you hear the surf? . . . Yes, I remembered to put on sun block."). Moreover, thanks to the advent of tiny headsets, even skiers on the slopes can transmit a second-by-second report of their progress ("You should be here! This is awesome! Whoa! Big mogul coming up! EEEEEEEK!")

The diabolical devices are everywhere. Nowhere are they more prevalent than in our institutions of learning, from colleges down to the elementary grades. It's highly unusual today to see a kid escaping from school at the end of the day who isn't talking on a cell phone. A child who doesn't have one is a social outcast, a pariah, a throwback to the Dark Ages. It won't be long before babies emerge from the womb clutching miniature cell phones to their tiny ears. And when the doctor smacks their bottoms, instead of crying, they'll yell, "Can you hear me now?"

I can understand the rationale: Parents believe they can keep track of their children by equipping them with cell phones. Yeah, right. As if when Mom calls, a kid is going to admit, "I'm at Susie's. Her parents aren't home so we're in her bedroom kicking back a few beers." Of course not. He'll say, "I'm just going into the library so gotta turn off my phone; I'll be home late. Got a ton of studying to do."

I was hoping that the advent of text messaging would at least reduce the number of ubiquitous conversations I'm forced to listen to everywhere, but no. It seems that senders of text messages are compelled to follow up with a voice call asking if the message was received. ("Did you get it? I sent it five minutes ago. No, not the one about my catching Jen in the sack with my brother—the one where I asked if you think I should get a second opinion before having a colonoscopy.")

Thank God he hadn't had the procedure yet. At least we were spared those details.

Do you know what I'm taking with me the next time I leave home? No, not my cell phone—industrial-strength ear plugs.

Just What the Doctor Ordered

I'm in love with my PCP. Not my personal computer pedagogue, my primary care physician. No, it's not what you think; my doctor is a woman. And, no, it's not what you're thinking now; I am not gay.

I love my lady doc because she has taken excellent care of me over the years. She's very thorough and is quick to refer me to specialists whenever she finds a potential problem. And when the problem is in my head, she's equally quick to dispense no-nonsense advice. For example, I have been very conscientious about walking briskly two miles a day; but after a couple of nasty falls caused by my clumsy stumbling, I told her I thought maybe I'd better stop walking. "Walk," she commanded. "Just pick up your feet." She's right. Her caveat now rings in my ear every time I set out.

Also, I've been worried about my cholesterol, which seemed high to me, according to what I've read. She pooh-poohed my fears saying that because my HDL/LDL ratio is excellent, the total number is fine. I sent my readings to another woman doctor, an e-mail friend in California. Her response, "This is a great profile. You're going to have to die at the hands of a jealous wife who finds you in bed with her husband. Listen to your doctor. She's right."

A while back, I attended a seminar on osteoporosis where doctors—and drug company representatives—painted a very bleak picture of what happens to women who do not take hormone replacements. We were all going to end up bent over double and with heart problems to boot. As for the possibility that hormones might promote any incipient breast cancer, that was a minor consideration, they said. Since I've had some borderline breast symptoms in the past, it was more than an insignificant matter for me. However, the heart issue was also a major concern since my mother and her siblings all had had serious cardiac problems. I asked my doctor what she thought.

"What do I think?" she replied. "I think you attend too many seminars."

She doesn't take hormones herself and very seldom recommends HRT, she said. A few days later, I read that a new study indicated that not only do hormones not help prevent heart problems, they may actually contribute to them. Again, my doctor was right. Of course, next week another group of researchers may disputes those findings, so everyone should consult with their own physicians before making any medical decisions. I know that I, for one, will continue to rely on my doctor.

And if I ever doubt her judgment, I just ask her for a second opinion from her mother. No, her mom is not a physician; but apparently she spends her days reading as many medical journals as she can get her hands on, and she passes the knowledge she gleans on to her daughter.

"Every night when I get home," says my doc, "I turn on my answering machine, and sure enough, there's at least one message from my mom. Last night it was, 'Judith, this is Mother. I was just reading that tomatoes are very beneficial for prostate problems; be sure to tell your male patients that they should eat as many tomato products as possible.'"

I think she should write a book titled *Judith, This Is Mother* and pass along all her mother's tips.

During my last annual exam, I asked Dr. Judy if it's true that one should take vitamin pills only with water.

"I don't know," she shrugged. "I take mine with coffee. Am I supposed to know that?"

"Look, do me a favor," I said. "Ask your mother."

I'm waiting for her to get back to me on that one. It may be a long wait. This relationship is not perfect, you see. My only complaint about my doctor is that though she gives me all the time I need during my annual physical exams, it's difficult to reach her by phone at other times. If I have a question, I have to ask her secretary who, in turn, relays it to my doctor or one of her nurses and then calls me back with an answer.

It's frustrating, but understandable; and it's not annoying enough to make me want to change doctors. After all, the next one might have a mother who just plays bridge all day.

Silly Science

Apparently, these days it's possible to shop for a designer baby as well as for designer clothes. A couple with big bucks who yearns for a perfect child can purchase an egg produced by the ovaries of a supermodel who is a member of Mensa; have it fertilized with sperm from a handsome Olympic gold medalist who is also a Pulitzer Prize-winning novelist; have the fertilized egg implanted into the womb of the wanna-be mom; and nine months later— voila! A gorgeous, gifted baby to call their own. Well, almost.

With designer babies in the offing, can designer pets be far behind? Apparently not. Felix Pets, a small company in Denver, Colorado, is developing allergen-free kittens for the one out of three cat owners in the United States who love their felines but are extremely sensitive to them. Before long, they may be able to purchase a nonsneeze-inducing cat at a price described only as "high," but the company's ultimate goal is to make the price "affordable."

Compared with these mind-boggling scenarios, the following recent scientific developments seem almost prosaic:

- Soon, moms may not be badgering their kids to drink their orange juice or take their vitamin pills. Instead, they'll nag, "Put on your vitamin C." They will not be talking about a new lotion, but about a T-shirt made from fiber containing a chemical developed by the Japanese firm Fuji Spinning Co. Ltd. This chemical responds to the warmth of human skin and turns into vitamin C, which is then absorbed into the body. Next on Fuji Spinning's drawing board is underwear infused with other vitamins. Fortunately, the clothing will be washable and its health-giving benefits estimated to survive thirty launderings.

• The next time you go to the grocery store, you may wonder why the packaged cheese is such a funny color. Because it's not cheese at all. It's peanut butter processed into slices and separated by waxed paper squares. That's one of the newest so-called advances in food technology developed by food processing engineers at the University of Oklahoma. Their goal? Convenience. God forbid Jimmy or Susie might have to open a jar and actually spread old-fashioned peanut butter onto a slice of bread. All that work would take away from their Nintendo time. In addition, it's much neater, has less chance of excess peanut butter getting trapped under the tongue stud, and is less likely to drip onto your vitamin C-infused T-shirt; therefore, it won't require an extra laundering, which would shorten its useful life. Of course, if Jimmy or Susie wants jelly with their PB, they'll have to do it the old fashioned way—at least for now. Jelly slices may already be in the works for all I know.

• Another innovation is the square watermelon developed by Japanese horticulturists. Sure they currently cost around $83.00, which is double or triple the price of a regular watermelon in Japan; but the cost is said to be worth the convenience of stacking the melons in the supermarket and storing them more easily in the fridge at home. What's next? Maybe rectangular turkeys that will fit nicely on the oven shelf? That would eliminate the Thanksgiving arguments over who gets the drumsticks. Where will it end?

• In France, they've already gone too far. A study of 34,000 French people supported the theory that "regular and moderate" consumption of red wine reduced the risks of cardiovascular disease by 30 percent. Fantastic news! We've been able to savor our dinner apéritif guilt-free, knowing it is therapeutic as well as enjoyable. Enter the French Distilleries Company to spoil it all by developing a pill to replace wine. Can you picture it? A romantic, candlelit dinner for two. He gazes into her eyes and proposes a toast, "To you, my precious chérie." She whispers, "No, mon amor. To us." Their eyes still locked, they pop pills, click their crystal water goblets, and sip. So maybe it's Perrier, but still . . . it's just not the same.

Don't you wonder what our great grandparents would say to all this? I never knew mine, but I can guess their reaction: "*Sono tutti pazzi!*" That's Sicilian for "They're all crazy!"

L'Antico, the Sicilian Confucius

Have you ever heard of l'Antico? His name, in lower case, means "the old man"; but with a capital "A," he's the Confucius of the Mediterranean—a Sicilian Chinese philosopher yet.

Of course, there were a few differences. Confucius was inscrutable, calm, wise; however, l'Antico, Mamma Mia! He was excitable, melodramatic, and emotional! (He was Sicilian, after all.) But he was also very wise—so wise that (if my relatives had been quoting him correctly for decades) he had something to say about every subject imaginable, even things that hadn't yet been thought of in his day. In fact, I have it on good authority (my Zia Maria) that l'Antico was the first proponent of trickle-down economics, which she claims was the real cause of the fall of the Roman Empire.

Hundreds of l'Antico's sayings have been handed down to us, in translation, almost word for word, including the mundane and familiar:

"Cani cc'abbaja no muzzica"—A barking dog doesn't bite.

"Ajutati ca' Dio t' ajuta"—God helps those who help themselves.

"A pignata vaddata, no n' vugghi mai"—A watched pot never boils.

Some of his other adages, on the other hand, convey familiar proverbs, but with a bit of a twist. Consider, for example, the following:

"*Sciumi ca grida assai, passalu sicuru/ Di sciumi mutu, passaci luntanu ma quannu grida passilu sicuru*"—You can pass a babbling brook safely. (Still waters run deep.)

"*Cu dommi, non pigghia pisci*"—He who sleeps doesn't catch any fish. (The early bird catches the worm.)

"*L'asinu e' ciecu e u patruni no n' vidi*"—The donkey is blind and the master can't see. (The blind leading the blind.)

"*Non si buttuni pi st'ucchjeddu*"—You're not a button for this buttonhole. (You can't put a square peg in a round hole.)

"*Cu accuzza, allonga*"—He who tries to shorten, lengthens. (Haste makes waste.)

Though we've been told that absence makes the heart grow fonder, l'Antico believed, "*L'avvicinamentu fa l'amuri,*" or proximity breeds love, which, come to think of it, is another way of saying "Out of sight, out of mind."

Still other of l'Antico's pearls of wisdom are either more inscrutable than anything ever attributed to Confucius or they lose something in the translation.

One example: "*Di jornu, ni ni vogghiu, e a sira spaddu l'ogghju,*" which means "During the day I don't want I, and at night I waste oil." Huh?

But he also had practical, easily comprehensible advice: "*Non sputari n' cjelu ca n' faccia ti torna,*" or "Don't spit in the sky because it will return to your face." Who can argue with such logic?

Because he was Italian, l'Antico had a different take on the grass always being greener in another person's yard. Instead, he observed that "*a mugghieri d'autru sempri pari chiu' bedda*" (Another's wife always seems more beautiful).

And no one who has ever heard it can forget the poignant, "*Passau du tempu ca Berta filava,*" or "The time for Bertha to weave is ended." Old timers say this is roughly equivalent to "Make hay while the sun shines," but it probably simply means that synthetic fibers and modern automated machinery have replaced the loom, so Bertha had better take a crash course in computer programming if she expects to find another job.

Speaking of jobs, l'Antico did not recommend multitasking. *"Cu assicuta dui cunigghi,"* he said, *"no n'afferra ne l' uno e ne l'autru,"* or "He who chases two rabbits will not catch either one."

And he also didn't ascribe to the "you can if you think you can" school of thought, since he preached, *"Cu auta a' pigghia, prestu si stocca,"* or *"Quantu e' chiu' grossa, chiu' presto si lassa,"* or *"The higher you reach, the faster you fall."*

Apparently human nature hasn't changed much since the days of l'Antico who said, *"Cu chiu' c' javi, chiu' assai voli,"* or "The more the rich man has, the more he wants." Frowning on greed, he advocated charitable sharing, warning, *"Cu mangja sulu s'affuca,"* or "He who eats alone, chokes."

Hundreds of other maxims—maybe even thousands—have been attributed to l'Antico.

Don't worry. I've forgotten the rest.

Those New Car Shopping Blues

Remember that old country song that warned mothers, "Don't let your babies grow up to be cowboys"? Well, better cowboys than car salesmen, I say. Actually, better cow *rustlers* than car salesmen.

But that may be unfair. After all, how can I compare? I've never met a cattle rustler nor have I ever had a cow rustled. In fact, I've never owned a cow. I have, however, owned several cars—some of which were overpriced, underperforming clunkers foisted on me by slick, high-pressure, promise-'em-everything desperados of the dealerships. Okay, to be fair, I admit I have known some very ethical car salesmen, but they're no fun to write about. So back to the scoundrels.

When I bought my last car, I knew exactly what I wanted— an economical, fuel-efficient four-cylinder with air conditioning. And, oh yes, it definitely had to be black. Instead, the salesman somehow talked me into an expensive, gas-guzzling six-cylinder. It was brown. It did not have air conditioning. But that was no problem, the salesman assured me. It's a fallacy, said he, that only factory-installed AC is satisfactory. They'd put in a system every bit as good. Better, even. And with the same warranty. He promised I'd love the car. He promised to drive me to work or lend me a car at no charge whenever mine needed servicing. He promised me thirty miles to the gallon in the city, despite the six cylinders. That did it. I signed on the dotted line. When I picked up my new car the following week, I tried to love it. I really did.

However, three days later, the air conditioner (which sounded like it should have been able to cool the Grand Canyon) gave up the fight. It emitted one last, terrible groan, threw up its fluid all over the floor, and died. I drove straight to the dealer. They were not happy to see me. Gone were the cheery smiles and firm handclasps of my previous visits. There was a definite chill in the air. Actually, it was a rather pleasant contrast to my automobile's steamy interior. Although they did not give me a warm reception, they did grudgingly agree to let me leave the car to be checked over. As for the ride to work or the loaner, however, what ride? What loaner? How could I possibly expect them to provide transportation for all their customers? Obviously, I had misunderstood. That was the high point. From there, it was all downhill. Even downhill, I got only fifteen miles to the gallon.

Never again would I be so gullible when buying a new car, I swore. But, then, I had made that same vow several times before and still managed to buy an array of motorized problems, instead of dependable transportation.

There was my new '76 Troubadour that refused to start whenever the temperature soared above fifty-five degrees or plummeted below forty-eight degrees, my '82 Gyro whose windshield leaked when it rained, my '89 Cruisemobile whose interior fogged up like a sauna as soon as I turned the ignition key, my '98 Tumbleweed whose brakes didn't . . .

What about warranties? Don't they mean anything? Of course they do. They guarantee you the right to park your new car, free of charge, in the dealer's garage whenever you have a problem. If they don't fix it, not to worry—just bring it in again . . . and again . . . and again. They'll take care of it this time for sure. That's a promise! Meanwhile, there you are trying to get home or to work. Have you ever tried driving a promise down the turnpike?

I recently decided to trade in my latest mistake. Its lifelong habit of lulling me into a false sense of security by performing beautifully for about five miles and then suddenly stalling when I slowed down in heavy traffic, with an eighteen-wheeler on my tail, had become too unnerving. I'm old. I've lost my sense of adventure.

Unfortunately, in order to have a new car, one must buy a new car; and in order to buy a new car, one must talk to new car salesmen. There's the rub.

Recalling all my prior unsuccessful forays to auto dealers, I ventured forth for a preliminary skirmish. Since all my previous lemons had rolled off Detroit assembly lines, I decided to investigate foreign automobiles. I went first to an Itsibitsi dealer. Charlie Charm greeted me at the threshold, shaking my hand with one of his, while holding the other out for a deposit.

"We're not getting another shipment for two months," he said. "If you don't put a deposit down today, the car you want could be gone tomorrow."

Since I had yet to form an emotional attachment for—or, in fact, even meet—any of his new cars, his threat was laughable. So I laughed. Charlie was confused. I was supposed to shake and quake and reach for my checkbook. Was something funny, he asked. Yes, I giggled. His high-pressure tactics. He excused himself and made a beeline for the back office. I made a beeline for the door. He was faster than I. Before I could escape, he returned with reinforcements—his manager, Larry Laidback, Mr. Low-Key himself. At least, that was the role he was playing in this particular charade.

Larry quickly assessed me as being a member of his generation, put on his sincere expression, and remarked what a pain "these hot-shot kids" can be, dismissing Charlie with a wave of his hand. Then he chuckled and started reminiscing about the good old days when we were kids, as though he and I had played Red Rover with the same gang under the street lamp in the old neighborhood. He didn't get around to the subject of cars for a good ten minutes; and at least three more minutes went by before he mentioned a deposit. He actually thought I was buying his act. This was no time for subtlety.

"Now that I've seen the car, I'm not interested," I said.

"Huh?" Larry didn't believe me. "Let me tell you what I can do for you . . ."

"Nothing will change my mind," I said. "Not even if you threw in a date with George Clooney."

He laughed heartily. "I like a woman with a good sense of humor," he said. "I'll just get the paperwork started while Charlie takes you for a test drive."

I definitely was not going to waste any time on a test drive. I bolted out the door and got as far as the curb, where I tripped over a small obstacle. It was an Itsibitsi. Charlie was holding its door open. I was trapped. He insisted I get behind the wheel, which was no easy feat. I felt as though I were going for a ride in Apollo 13.

"Gee, there's not much room, is there?" I observed.

"How about that stereo!" said Charlie, turning up the volume.

I told him if there was anything I hated more than high-pressure salesmanship, it was high-volume stereo. He couldn't hear me.

"Turn left here," he yelled.

To his dismay, I turned right. The road sloped gently upward. The Itsibitsi gasped and wheezed as it struggled to keep going.

"It doesn't have much power, does it?" I asked.

"Some stereo, huh?" grinned Charlie, turning the volume louder still.

I headed back to the dealership.

"You're really lucky," said Charlie as I tried to squeeze out from behind the steering wheel. "This is the last one on the lot in this color."

Even if I absolutely loved the car, the color—a bilious green—would have killed the deal. And I did not absolutely love the car.

Larry was lounging against the door waiting for me. "Good

news!" he said. "I've been working the numbers, and I can let you have that beauty for a rock-bottom price. Only $28,900, plus your trade-in!"

I was speechless. "It's okay," he beamed. "You don't have to thank me. Now, do you want thirty-six months or forty-eight months financing?"

"Neither," I managed to spit out through clenched teeth.

"Smart move," he replied. "If we spread it over sixty months, the payments will be a breeze. Now let's see," he said, turning his back to pick up his calculator. "That will come to . . ."

I made a dash for the door, ran out, jumped into my car, and gunned the motor.

"Please," I begged it. "Don't stall now. Wait for an eighteen-wheeler."

"Stop!" Larry called. "Let's talk. That price is negotiable."

I pulled away from the curb just as he reached me.

"28,500," he yelled . . . "27,900 . . . 27,500 . . ." His voice faded away as I drove off.

I looked in my rear-view mirror. Larry had stumbled and fallen into the gutter. Right where he belonged.

The Woes of the Single Humor Writer

Every trade has its tools. For a humor writer, the three most important requirements are a sense of the absurd, a computer or word processor, and a spouse—not necessarily in that order. Though the first two are key, without the last one, a humorist is truly handicapped. Not only are mates a treasure trove of comic ideas just by themselves, they can also provide children, who are an endless source of hilarity (as long as you keep that aforementioned sense of the absurd).

For instance, do you think Erma Bombeck (whose writing I always loved) would have made the splash she did if she had been single, like me? Don't get me wrong. She was a clever, talented lady; but in addition to her natural wit, she had two huge advantages—a husband and kids. In other words, a live-in cast of characters feeding her material and dialogue daily.

Erma had it made from the day she said, "I do." Even before, as a matter of fact. If she had been writing back then, she could have done a whole series of articles on the wedding alone: Drawing up the guest list ("I don't see why we can't invite my uncle Rocky; he'll be out on parole by then."); choosing the bridesmaids ("I know you're my best friend, Clarabelle; but you'll be eight-and-a-half-months pregnant, and I don't want to be upstaged by the stork."); planning the reception ("I realize that pheasant is expensive, Daddy; but I'll die if we have to serve peanut butter sandwiches."); the mishaps during the ceremony (the best man losing the ring, the groom losing his lunch, the organist losing her music and playing the only song she knew from memory, "Please Release Me."); the departure for the honeymoon amid tears and hysterics (the groom's mother's).

His mother would also come in handy when the honeymoon was over to provide all the standard meddling mother-in-law humor. Then there could be tales of learning-to-cook disasters, the first quarrel, the division of household chores disputes, the disagreements about whose parents to visit for the holidays . . .

And when those wells ran dry, all Erma had to do was get pregnant—a surefire source of material for daily columns for nine months. It's always hysterical to read about someone else's morning sickness. As for labor and delivery, they're a scream.

Then, of course, there's the baby itself and its comically adorable and/or humorously aggravating progress from infancy to the terrible twos through the terrifying teens. If Erma needed an idea for Monday's column, she could merely peek into the bedlam of her son's bedroom and get enough inspiration for every Monday of the year. On Tuesday, she could always rely on her husband to say or do something hopelessly unromantic or chauvinistic, and a thousand words would be a snap. On Wednesday, she merely had to look into the washing machine where she would be sure to find a hitherto missing pet frog, the family cat humorously frazzled, the cake she had baked for the church fair, and three unmated (like me) socks. On Thursday, her little girl might decide that her twelve Barbie dolls would like to go for a swim—in the toilet bowl. The resulting clog would necessitate a visit from a plumber who would turn out to be a Jay Leno clone; and quotes from him would help her meet her deadlines for the rest of the week.

If things ever got dull around the house, Erma could simply go to a PTA meeting, and the teacher's tales of Junior's antics would supply enough material for a year's worth of columns.

I, on the other hand, don't have all those people helping me since I foolishly never realized the commercial value of a husband and children, and I remained single. That wouldn't be bad if I were a twenty-year-old swinger and could mesmerize readers with anecdotes about my hedonistic lifestyle. Once, when I was younger, I did try to join one of those couples swap clubs advertised on the Internet, purely for research purposes, of course; but they refused me membership when they investigated and found out about me. Not that I'm a writer, but that I didn't have a mate to swap.

Unfortunately, I never find zany surprises in my washing machine; and though I do need to call a repairman from time to time, instead of Jay Leno I usually get Solemn Sam. I did crash a PTA meeting once, pretending to be a parent, but I couldn't pull it off. I didn't look harried enough.

I once even tried one of Erma's old tricks of wearing ankle socks with my wedgies. She always got hysterical reactions when she did that. Regrettably, my timing was off. I waited too long, and all I got was admiration for being one of the first to wear a kicky new fashion.

I guess if I want to get serious about my humor, though it's a bit late, I'm going to have to get myself a husband. I'm holding auditions next Monday from 10:00 A.M. to 4:00 P.M. All applicants will be judged on witty repartee and appearance. Neatness does *not* count since there's nothing funny about unrumpled socks and shoes that match. Ad libbers who don't use prepared notes will be given preference, as will applicants with domineering mothers. Oh, wait. That ship has sailed. It's not likely that applicants my age have mothers who are still living. I will therefore settle for someone with an obnoxious, intrusive ex-wife and/or dysfunctional grandchildren.

Who am I kidding? At this point, I will consider anyone who inhales and exhales fairly regularly.

Friendship

Sally and I are great friends, though it's hard to understand why. We have so little in common.

Sally is happiest when she's behind the wheel of her car. Her idea of a good time is a long ride, which is my idea of torture.

"Let's go to lunch," she'll say.

Why not? Sounds good to me. Next thing I know we're heading to a mountain-top inn 120 miles from home. I was thinking more in terms of that new sandwich shop on the next block.

She loves to listen to music while driving—oldies, new age, whatever. Talk radio is my choice (except for commentators who don't share my political views).

And guess who else disagrees with my politics? That's right. Sally.

I hate to shop. She loves it. She swears she doesn't, but a "Sale" or "Outlets" sign draws her car like a magnet.

I enjoy almost all movies and the theater indiscriminately. Sally doesn't. I think I know why. She can't abide sitting in one spot for a couple of hours—time that could be spent aimlessly driving somewhere.

Having grown up with two brothers, Sally is a sports fan. She loves to watch baseball, football, hockey, basketball, track, NASCAR—anything but figure skating. Can you guess which is the only sport I (a sibling-deprived child) enjoy watching? Yep, I love those spins . . . jumps . . . axles . . . lutzes . . . salchows. I can't tell one from the other, but I find them all mesmerizing.

When Sally watches sports—or anything—on TV, she constantly surfs from channel to channel. It drives me crazy! Pick a show and keep it there, for heaven's sake! I have to take a Dramamine before watching television at her house.

We do both enjoy travel and have taken many trips together. I prefer a fixed itinerary. Not Sally, of course. She abhors being tied to a particular schedule. And while I much prefer to fly to a destination more than a few hundred miles away, Sally would rather drive—again, the schedule phobia, and also because her car has a huge trunk that she can pack with every article of clothing she has owned since college and still have room for all the treasures she'll buy along the way. I'm happier with having to keep track of only what will fit in one small suitcase; and since there's no room to spare (and since I'm basically a tightwad), I'm better able to resist any impulsive purchases that I know I'll regret when I return home.

Unlike most of our other friends, Sally and I do have a love of gadgets in common, especially electronic thingamajigs. We've both had computers since floppy disks actually were floppy (remember those?) and can spend hours on the phone trying to help each other when we can't figure out how to make our PCs do what we want them to.

Sally is far more selfless than I. She constantly rushes to help whichever friend within a thousand-mile radius has broken an ankle, sprained a back, or come down with the flu—even if she hasn't yet had her own flu shot. Me, I'm a hypochondriac (and probably basically lazy); I stay away. And she always finds the flimsiest excuses to shower people with lavish gifts. (Me? See "tightwad" reference above.)

I sold my house several years ago and bought a condo, the eighth move of my life. I could not be bothered with all those home maintenance responsibilities, either doing them myself or finding someone to take care of them—mowing the lawn, trimming the shrubs, weeding the garden, painting the shutters, repairing the roof, repaving the driveway, fixing the dripping faucets, shoveling snow off the walk . . . the list was endless and daunting. Sally, however, who was born in the house where she still lives and does not intend to move in the foreseeable future, thrives on what I consider all that drudgery. How she finds the time, I can't imagine since she's still working part time. Is it any surprise to learn that I couldn't wait to retire?

Sally is a very private person, whereas I am apt to blab every detail of my life—and maybe yours. Well, not really. At least I'd like to think I'd keep your secrets. But with Sally, there's no doubt whatsoever. If you tell her something in confidence, even the threat of hanging wouldn't get her to reveal it.

Despite her many admirable attributes, she does have a flaw or two, one of which is her chronic tardiness. It's not that she doesn't leave her house in time for any appointments. It's just that she always seems to have errands to run on the way. She has to go to the bank, the grocery store, the dry cleaner, the drug store, and she never seems to calculate how much time these detours will eat up. I must say, though, she's been getting much better about this lately, which is very disconcerting. Because I always assume she'll be late, I take my time; and Sally ends up waiting for me.

We do share the same basic values and the same religion (though I'm much more critical of it than she is).

Sally truly is a beautiful person (unlike the "beautiful people" who bug me), and I believe that associating with her has made me a finer human being. What better qualification for friendship can there be?

By the way, Sally isn't her real name. She'd be very embarrassed if I revealed her identity. (See—I *can* keep a secret!)